What people are saying about Katy Gordon and the book:

"There is a lot that each of us can do to stay healthy. High blood pressure is a major risk factor for heart disease and stroke, and is a very common condition. If you have high blood pressure it is important that you know as much as possible about it, learn to live with it and manage it yourself. This book provides you with the wherewithal to do this. If you look after your body it will look after you."

— Sir Ranulph Fiennes

"Katy Gordon is an amazing leader with a huge heart and passion for helping her patients and clients to live a healthier and more fulfilling life packed with more energy, less stress and more control of what has become a silent killer in our society. What price can you put on good health? I would say far more than the cost of this wonderful book so take your copy home today. You'll be glad you did."

— Paul "Turbo Coach" Avins
Founder of The Business Wealth Club

"Katy Gordon has written a complete resource guide to self managment of high blood pressure. The book covers everything in an easy to understand format that really works. I would recommend it to anyone who is serious about beating this deadly disease or simply wants to maintain a high standard of health. I can't think of a single person who wouldn't benefit from the information Katy provides. If you value your health, you need to read this book and take action!"

— Chelsey Baker, Journalist

"This is a book for patients, written by a patient who also has a large background in nursing. It has up to date good advice about what patients should do about treatment in order to lower their blood pressure."

— The Blood Pressure Association

GW00670974

1

"I just assumed that this was how the rest of life was going to be, and, although I was only in my mid-forties, I began to resign myself to the prospect of being a semi-invalid for the coming years. My business partner, though, felt certain that there was something wrong which could be put right, with the appropriate expert help and advice. She introduced me to Katy Gordon.

Katy immediately made me feel much better, by reassuring me that there was clearly something wrong with my pacemaker, and that what was needed was for it to be sorted out, and that certainly I did not need to resign myself to a sedentary life. I made an appointment to see my hospital consultant. Katy spoke to him as well, and was able to discuss matters with him with knowledge and understanding. As a result of this consultation, and the clarity which Katy had been able to provide, the consultant decided that I needed a new pacemaker and associated wires.

I duly had the operation, but, while it went well surgically, I was no better in myself. I built up my running slowly – to just three miles – but felt completely exhausted and couldn't build it up further. I was also waking up in the morning with no energy and feeling really sluggish again.   In despair I rang Katy again. She was wonderfully reassuring. She said I probably needed a 'box check', but that, before contacting the technician, she would like to understand just what I was looking for. It was probably unlikely that I would still be able to undertake the same kind of physical activities I had enjoyed in my twenties, or even in my thirties. So what did I want to achieve? "To be able to run five or ten miles without feeling knackered," I immediately replied. "Fine," said Katy. "Now we've got a clear goal."

Katy spoke to the technician, and explained that my pacemaker seemed to reach a ceiling when my heart rate increased to a certain level but I felt there was more to give. She explained what I wanted to be able to do, and asked him to check the 'pacing threshold' and to increase the maximum heart rate the pacemaker was set to.

Because Katy had been able to explain my symptoms to the technician in language she could understand, she was able to reset my pacemaker to match my needs. And now not only can I run ten miles without collapsing – last October I ran the Loch Ness marathon in 3hrs 36 minutes! Not bad for a 50 year old! My latest pacing check has confirmed everything is working fine and it was a fantastic feeling being able to show the cardiac technician my certificate for completing the Loch Ness marathon. I would never have believed I would be considering my next marathon in the lovely New Forest without Katy's support.

My transformation from despairing exhaustion to renewed energy and zest for life is entirely down to Katy. Her combination of medical expertise, sensitive questioning and clear communication meant that I was able to receive the treatment I needed, effectively and without a fuss. I am eternally grateful to Katy for giving me back my quality of life."

— GR, SE England

BEATING HIGH BLOOD PRESSURE

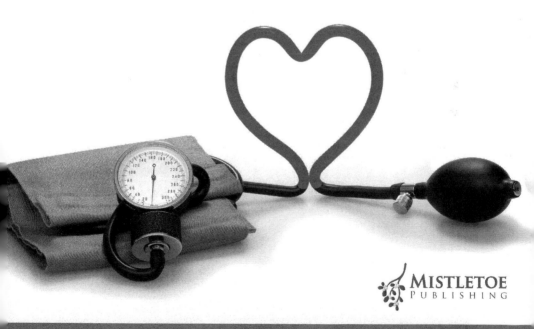

MISTLETOE
PUBLISHING

KATY GORDON

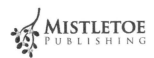

Beating High Blood Pressure
Katy Gordon

Published 2011
Mistletoe Publishing
3 Belmont Hill
Newport
Essex
CB11 3RF

ISBN 978-0-9568635-0-8

Cover, design, illustrations and typesetting by www.sunmakers.co.uk
Typeset in Minion Pro and Gill Sans.
Printed in Great Britain by Short Run Press ltd.

www.katygordon.com

✚ Dedication

This book has been through many iterations, and it has been touch and go as to whether it would actually get published. I am delighted to say that it now has finally come to fruition with the help and support of some people who are very dear to me. Without their very much appreciated help and support this book would not have happened.

Huge thanks go to Sarah for her incredible skills with words and her knowledge of the publishing world.
She has always been there with words of encouragement and support and has worked her magic with her editing skills too.

Another big thank you goes to my good friend and business mentor, Paul. He has always had faith in my abilities and cajoled, encouraged or pushed me depending on what I needed at the time. Without him and Sarah this book would not be here.

My sister, Tammy, has also given me valuable support and help with the proof reading as well as with words of encouragement and cups of tea along the way.

Megan has also been a huge help with editing the earlier drafts, and with giving some very good suggestions which are included in the book – thank you! Thanks also go to Elizabeth who helped me with the exercise section.

I would also like to thank the staff who work during the afternoons at the Cricketers in Clavering, as they provided me with pots of tea and occasionally a slice of delicious cake to nourish my brain while I wrote the more difficult parts in this book.

The other people who have all helped to make this book happen are the colleagues and patients I have worked with throughout all my clinical experience and who are the unsung heroes of this book. They are the people who treated or had high blood pressure, who have taught me so much and are also the inspiration behind the book.

My friend, Damian, has sent me two short articles at the end of the Psychological Wellbeing section which I think really enhances that section. He whistled them up in a trice too, a big thank you to him.

Finally I would like to dedicate this book to all those of you out there who either have high blood pressure, or want to know more about high blood pressure for whatever the reason. I hope this book gives you what you need to make the right choices for you, so that you can live your life to the full, stay healthy and enjoy it!

Katy Gordon, 2011

✚ Contents

Part 1: **Everything you need to know about your blood pressure**

Part 2: **What you can do to help yourself**

Part 3: **My Blood Pressure Action Plan**

List of Illustrations

Foreword

High blood pressure is a major risk for important diseases of the circulation such as heart attack, stroke and chronic kidney disease. The condition is very common and, because many people are unaware that they have a problem, it often goes untreated.

In fact, blood pressure management is better in the United Kingdom than in most other countries but there is a long way to go before we get to an optimal position.

Stroke is a particular risk relating to high blood pressure. This horrific process is often regarded as an inevitable consequence of old age but in reality, one in four of all cases affect people under the age of sixty-five.

There is a great deal that individuals can do to reduce their own blood pressure and this something that all of us can do to help ourselves regardless of whether or not our own blood pressure is high. The first is to lead a healthy life that, in this context, means taking regular exercise, eating a healthy diet and minimising the amount of salt in our diet. Unfortunately, today many foods contain much more salt than is necessary and consumers have to work quite hard to ensure that they do not exceed their normal daily requirement.

This is why I am happy to recommend this text to the reader. It is vital that people who have high blood pressure, as I do myself, know as much as possible about their condition and, as far as is possible, learn to manage the condition themselves.

The average blood pressure for people in the UK has fallen over recent years largely through better identification and better treatment provided by excellent health professionals. But it is the individual who lives with the condition, it is the individual who has to live with the prospect of taking tablets for many years and it is the individual who has to live with the consequences should things go wrong. It is essential then that individuals do all they can to manage their condition themselves and aspire to help their professional advisers to help them to do this.

That is why I recommend this text to a wide audience. It might be your turn next.

Professor Roger Boyle CBE
National Director for Heart Disease and Stroke
Department of Health

London, December 2010

+ Introduction

The management of long-term conditions such as high blood pressure has been a part of my everyday working life for the past 25 and more years. I want to share with you what I know to be the most effective way of managing the condition and show you how to be healthier as a result. I have gained my knowledge over the years, based on learning from those who have been and are living with high blood pressure, and also from working with various highly skilled, knowledgeable and expert healthcare professionals - doctors, nurses, pharmacists etc.

High blood pressure is a condition which you and I can do a lot to manage effectively ourselves even if we need to take medication for it. Increasingly people at a younger age are developing it. The Labour government, in 2008, set out plans to identify people who are at risk of developing cardiovascular disease, including high blood pressure, which they wanted to see systematically implemented from April 2009. In theory this is a fantastic idea, but sadly in practice it discriminates against younger people because they put a lower age limit for these health checks to happen. As a result younger adults under the age of 40 are not eligible to have a health check done. This is such a missed opportunity as it means that quite a large number of people will not have diagnoses such as high blood pressure, high cholesterol levels, or diabetes diagnosed until they develop a problem with it. This is such a crying shame as there is so much that can be done for these various conditions which can reduce or prevent problems arising if they are diagnosed early enough. Therefore the tranche of people under the age of 40 who fall into this category will be disadvantaged as a result. As the public becomes more aware of the potential seriousness of having high blood pressure they can do more themselves to prevent it happening.

I myself have high blood pressure, diagnosed more recently, and have had to learn to manage it.

The book is split into three parts:

Part 1 covers the basics that you need to know about your condition. All the answers to the questions you wish you had asked when still with your doctor, but didn't ask because you were busy taking on board your diagnosis. Once you know exactly what you are dealing with it is much easier to manage and to formulate a plan to move forward with your life.

Part 2 looks at what you can do to help yourself. This section lists the changes that can be made to your lifestyle that will help you become fitter, healthier and in control of your own health. It is all too easy to feel out of control when you have a new diagnosis and this book aims to give you back that control.

Throughout the book an easy-to-use traffic light system will guide you in helping yourself and also help you decide when you need to go and see a medical professional to check your symptoms and advise you individually. I have also provided sensible advice on leading a healthy lifestyle to reduce your risk of developing further problems.

Prevention is always better than cure and usually much less painful.

Part 3 is a personal action plan for you to fill in so that you can monitor your own progress at home..

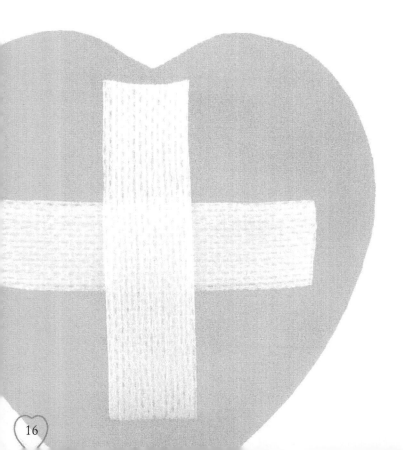

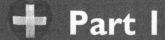

Part I

Everything you need to know about your blood pressure

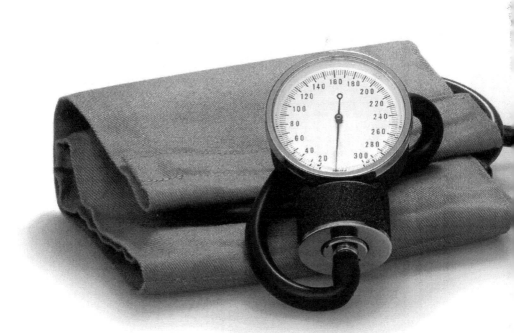

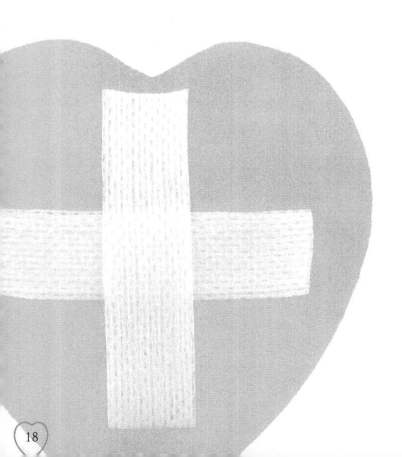

What can I do if I have high blood pressure?

Millions of people live with long-term conditions such as high blood pressure. Most of these people lead a full and active life by adapting their lifestyles in response to their condition. By increasing your understanding of your condition and how you can help yourself to health, you can improve the quality of your life. High blood pressure should be regarded as a warning sign for other more serious conditions (such as heart and kidney disease, diabetes and stroke) so it is well worth taking note of the things you can do to improve your health if you are diagnosed with it.

Some facts about high blood pressure:

▶ 16 million people in the UK have high blood pressure

▶ 130,000 people in the UK have a stroke every year, which is about 1 person every 5 minutes

▶ 1 in 3 with high blood pressure don't know that they have got it

---

A long-term condition affects your health over a long period of time, possibly your entire life and in many cases, there is no cure. When you are first diagnosed it is easy to feel overwhelmed and as if the condition has taken over your life. This can be especially so if you need to take medication – drugs or pills - on a daily basis or have to monitor your blood pressure. It is important to understand, though, that your condition can become a serious problem. But, there is a lot you can do to help counteract and control the negative effects on your health.

One method of taking control is "self-management." Believe this, and start getting motivated to make the changes to your lifestyle and engage in active self management. When you take care of your body, it will take care of you and prevent problems in the future.

What is blood pressure?

This is the pressure of the blood in your circulation or arteries. The blood in the arteries is very important as it carries all the vital nutrients (absorbed mainly through your gut) and oxygen (from the lungs) to the tissues in your body. This is essential to maintain the body's day-to-day working functions. Blood, once in your veins, is empty of the nutrients and oxygen and is on its way back to the heart and lungs for more. On the way back it removes the waste products of metabolism (such as carbon dioxide) from the tissues to the organs (for instance, the liver and the kidneys), where they are processed and then eliminated from the body. This whole system of arteries, veins and capillaries (the tiny blood vessels close to the surface of the skin) is known generally as your circulation system.

In order for the blood to get around your body, your heart pumps the blood out into the arteries or 'arterial' system. If the blood is to get to all the different parts of your body a reasonable pressure must be maintained. When the heart contracts to pump blood out through the arteries your blood pressure goes up, and when the heart relaxes it goes down.

The Circulatory System

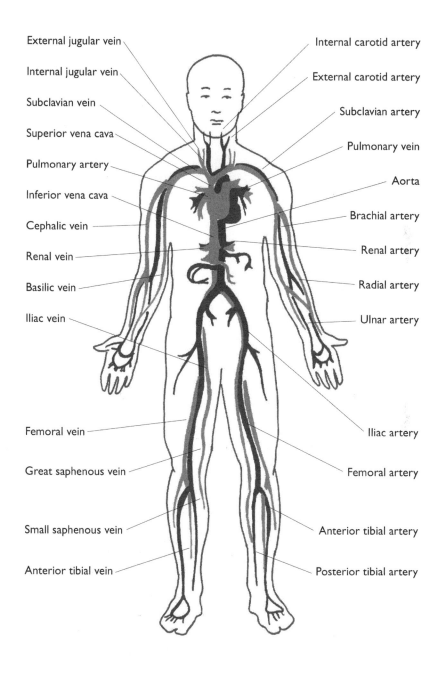

External jugular vein

Internal jugular vein

Subclavian vein

Superior vena cava

Pulmonary artery

Inferior vena cava

Cephalic vein

Renal vein

Basilic vein

Iliac vein

Femoral vein

Great saphenous vein

Small saphenous vein

Anterior tibial vein

Internal carotid artery

External carotid artery

Subclavian artery

Pulmonary vein

Aorta

Brachial artery

Renal artery

Radial artery

Ulnar artery

Iliac artery

Femoral artery

Anterior tibial artery

Posterior tibial artery

This is your 'blood pressure' – the difference in pressure between your heart contracting and relaxing.

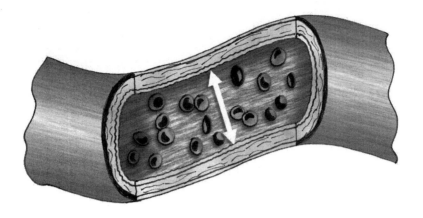

Blood pressure is the measurement of force applied to the artery wall

What is normal blood pressure?

When your blood pressure is measured two numbers are taken. They are written down by doctors and nurses as if they are a mathematical fraction, such as 130/80 mmHg. The measure of a mercury column, taken in millimetres of mercury (mmHg), is how blood pressure is usually taken in the UK. The top number, which you may hear called the *systolic* pressure, tells you the pressure in your arteries when the heart is pumping blood to go to all the different parts of the body. The lower or second number is called the *diastolic* pressure, shows the pressure in your arteries when the heart is resting in between beats. If you have your blood pressure taken abroad it may be measured in kilopascals (kPa) which are part of the International System of measurement (SI units)

What should my blood pressure be?

The top number, or systolic, should normally be between 90 – 140 mmHg, ideally no higher than 120 mmHg, but can be anything up to 240 mmHg. The lower number, or diastolic, should be anywhere between 60 – 90 mmHg, ideally no higher than 80 mmHg, but could be anything up to 140 mmHg. The only way of measuring your blood pressure is to have it taken using a sphygmomanometer. Your doctor or nurse may use either a manual or electronic machine. In either case, they involve placing a material 'cuff' around your upper arm, with the cuff being first inflated and then deflated, a bit like a balloon. Throughout the day it is normal to have changes in your blood pressure, both up and down, linked to things such as physical activity or rest etc. This is normal! However sustained high blood pressure is not.

What is high blood pressure?

This is when the pressure in the system is higher than it should be. It is also called *hypertension*. If this higher pressure continues for a long time it can damage some of your vital organs by putting a strain on the arteries carrying blood to, and within them. Because of the strain, or increased persistent pressure, these arteries can become weakened or they can become clogged up with fatty deposits (also called atheroma) which in turn can lead to narrowing of these arteries. This can then result in clots forming in the arteries, causing a blockage, which can cause subsequent damage to the organ. The two most vulnerable organs for this to occur in are the heart and brain, although other parts of the body including the kidneys, hands and legs can become affected too. The most common conditions to occur as a result of this are heart attacks or angina, and strokes or mini strokes (also called transient ischaemic attacks, or TIAs).

Because of the added pressure in the system this puts added strain on your heart which has to pump the blood through these narrowed arteries.

There is another medical condition that can be caused by having high blood pressure, especially if it is not well treated and managed at an early stage. This condition is called heart failure and it comes about because your heart has to work consistently harder to pump blood around the body. It can also happen after a heart attack, due to the damage caused to the heart muscle. If this happens for a prolonged period of time the heart stops pumping as well as it has done in the past. Basically it gets a bit tired, like any muscle, but it does not get an opportunity to have a rest as other muscles do. Over a period of time of not pumping as well as it should, you may feel tired and a bit short of breath, you may also notice your ankles swell too. You may start to notice it more at particular times of day, or when doing particular daily activities. You may also feel that you are just a bit unfit and that you are getting older. Because of this, it may be difficult for your doctor to know that you have got some heart failure unless you describe your symptoms to them carefully.

If your blood pressure becomes too high you also increase your risk of developing other medical conditions compared to people who do not have raised blood pressure. This can cause damage to some of your vital organs. Having high blood pressure increases your risk of developing heart disease or stroke, although there are other things called risk factors which can also increase your risk. This is often known as an increased risk of developing cardiovascular disease – literally 'heart and stroke' disease. We discuss what this means later on in the book.

Having a chronically high blood pressure means you are more likely to develop one or more of the following later on in your life:

- heart disease – angina and heart attacks
- strokes and mini strokes,
- heart failure
- kidney damage or disease
- kidney stones and osteoporosis
- eye problems
- stomach cancer
- dementia

It is important to try and prevent your level of risk becoming high and this can be done in several different ways. Risk factors and how to have your level of risk assessed are discussed later in this book. Please see page 37

What causes persistent or sustained high blood pressure?

For most people, their blood pressure is not due to any definite cause. Doctors call this *essential hypertension* - this is when the small blood vessels in the body narrow, causing pressure to build up. If you imagine a garden hose being squeezed, it is a similar effect to what happens in your body. There are a few people who get what is known as *secondary hypertension*, which is when you get high blood pressure due to something else going on in your body. This can happen if you get some problems with your kidneys, or also the adrenal glands, which sit on top of the kidneys, and produce hormones which help to control your blood pressure. If there is a problem with your adrenal glands it may only become apparent when you have your blood pressure taken and it is found to be quite high.

Sometimes women can get high blood pressure when they're pregnant. If this happens the medical staff will want to keep a close eye on it and will ask you to rest and take things very easy. You may hear this referred to as a condition called *pre-eclampsia*. If the blood pressure stays high it can become quite serious, in other words it progresses, so it is very important to follow your doctor's advice. You may be admitted to hospital for strict bed rest to help stop it getting any higher. Less frequently the doctors may decide you need to have a Caesarean section – in other words they do an operation to get the baby born so that both your and the baby's health are not put in any further danger. Usually, once the baby is born, your blood pressure will go back to normal. If you get pregnant again and have already had this condition, pre-eclampsia, the doctors will keep a much closer eye on you from early on in your pregnancy to try and prevent it happening again, or at the very least to alert them quickly if you do start to develop it.

Is high blood pressure common?

High blood pressure is quite common in the UK. One out of three adults now has it, and it is more common in people in older age groups. In the UK approximately 16 million people have a blood pressure above 140/90mmHg.

Have I got high blood pressure?

If you have high blood pressure you are *unlikely to have any signs or symptoms.* This is the main reason why you may not know that you have high blood pressure. You may have seen references in the press to the 'silent killer' and this is what high blood pressure is sometimes referred to as. The only way to know if you have high blood pressure or not is to have it measured, which is why it is so important to have it checked regularly.

For this reason it is very important that you have your blood pressure checked regularly as you get older. You may be feeling absolutely fine and have no idea that you have high blood pressure. In years gone by it was often only when someone had a stroke or mini stroke that they were diagnosed as having high blood pressure. Regular blood pressure checks could stop this happening to you.

Regular health checks are a good idea. Your car needs to have regular checks once a year when it has an MOT. Doing the same for your body is exactly the same idea although it is not something many people do on a regular basis. Think of it as your own body's MOT and remember to go and see your general practice team at least once every five years for a health check until you reach middle age and then more frequently, unless you see them about something else more regularly. As part of your health check it is always a good idea to know what your numbers are especially in relation to your blood pressure and cholesterol levels. The Blood Pressure Association, a national charity, holds a *Know Your Numbers* week every September as part of a campaign to support you to know more about what your blood pressure is and how important it is to make sure your blood pressure is normal. During this week thousands of blood pressure tests are offered free throughout the UK – your local surgery should have details of where and how you can get your blood pressure tested as part of this campaign, or alternatively look on the Association's website (see the 'useful websites' information on page 161) for details of where it is available locally to you.

Is high cholesterol related to high blood pressure?

You may also want to have your cholesterol checked regularly too. As with high blood pressure, high cholesterol does not always have any symptoms so it is a good idea to get your cholesterol levels checked too.

Cholesterol is a fatty, slightly waxy substance which is produced by the liver from the saturated fats that we eat. It plays a vital role in cell function, and also production of hormones and Vitamin D. Once it has done its job in the body, it is also the liver's job to break it down and get rid of the excess from the body. This is what happens in normal healthy people as part of our body functioning properly. The liver has finger-like receptors which reach out and grab the 'bad' particles of cholesterol, also known as LDL, as they pass, and then breaks down the excess.

We also have another type of cholesterol which is the 'good' type, and is also known as HDL cholesterol. The good HDL cholesterol travels through the arteries and helps unblock them, before it too returns to the liver and is also broken down by another set of receptors, and removed from the body. Once cholesterol is inside the liver it gets broken down and travels down the bile duct into the intestines, or gut, where it is passed out of the body and excreted with the remains of the digested food.

The most common reason for high cholesterol is because we have too much of the LDL or 'bad' cholesterol for our receptors to cope with. Over the course of time cholesterol builds up in the arteries and deposits of cholesterol restrict the blood flow, causing a narrowing of the artery. This increases your risk of having a heart attack or stroke. In some people the artery blocks off completely causing severe chest pain and a heart attack.

Some people can have a very high cholesterol level because they have what is called Familial Hypercholesterolaemia, which literally means a high cholesterol or lipid level which runs in the family and is passed on in the genes. These people can have bad angina, on indeed a heart attack, at a much younger age, some as young as in their 30s or 40s. If there are no warning signs it is not very easy to tell if you should be checked over by your family doctor/GP. If you do have a high cholesterol it is always a good idea to ask other directly related members of your family to get their cholesterol levels checked too, in case they have a raised cholesterol and need to be treated too.

Who is likely to get high blood pressure?

Anyone can get high blood pressure but some people are more likely to develop it. These groups of people include:

- Someone who has a family history of high blood pressure, stroke or heart attack. In other words if your mother or father or a close family relative has had any of these conditions you are more likely to develop it yourself.

- Some other conditions which you may already have which are closely linked to having high blood pressure. These include diabetes, heart disease and kidney disease. So if you have any of these diseases it is very important that you have your blood pressure checked regularly, and if you are then discovered to have high blood pressure, that it is kept under control.

- People from some specific ethnic groups are more likely to have high blood pressure. If you are black you are more likely to have high blood pressure than the rest of the population in the UK. You may also be more sensitive to salt in your diet and also more likely to have a stroke. Salt can have quite an effect on your blood pressure so it is a good idea to be careful how much salt you add to your food. This is discussed in more detail later in this book on page 37. South Asians are more likely to have diabetes or a heart attack or angina. If you are South Asian it is important for you to keep not only your blood pressure but also your cholesterol levels under control and within normal limits. The reasons for this are not fully understood but the links are definitely there.

Normal values for blood pressure and cholesterol levels

Cholesterol and Triglyceride Levels for People without Heart Disease, mmol/l

Blood Lipid	Good	Borderline	High
Total cholesterol	< 4 or less	4 - 5	> 5
LDL cholesterol ("bad cholesterol")	< 2 or less	2 - 3	> 3
Triglycerides	< 2		
HDL cholesterol ("good cholesterol")	Male: 0.9 -1.4 Female: 1.2 -1.7		

Blood Pressure Levels for People without Heart Disease or Diabetes, mmHg

Blood Pressure	Good	Normal	Borderline	High
Systolic (when the heart contracts and pumps blood out.)	120 or less	120-140	141-160	160 and higher
Diastolic (between beats, as your heart rests and fills with blood again.)	70 or less	70--85	86--90	91 and higher

Blood Pressure Levels for People without Heart Disease but **with Diabetes,** mmHg

Blood Pressure	Good	Normal	Borderline	High
Systolic (when the heart contracts and pumps blood out.)	120 or less	120-130	131-140	140 and higher
Diastolic (between beats, as your heart rests and fills with blood again.)	70 or less	70--80	80--85	86 and higher

Your lifestyle can affect not only your blood pressure but your cholesterol levels too. You are much more likely to have high blood pressure if you:

- eat a lot of salt
- drink a lot of alcohol
- don't eat enough fibre in your diet i.e. fruit and vegetables
- are overweight
- are not physically active
- smoke (even socially)
- have too much stress in your life

You will find more information on your recommended daily allowances in the second part of the book.

Having a healthy lifestyle helps reduce your likelihood of having high blood pressure, as well as reducing your risk of developing heart disease or stroke. You can make relatively easy changes to your lifestyle and reduce your risk. I will talk about what you can do to become healthier in the next part of the book.

What about STRESS?

Research evidence is beginning to recognise that, for some people, prolonged episodes of stress may contribute to high blood pressure. We cannot measure stress easily which makes this area quite complex to research. However, stress can affect the heart by releasing certain chemicals or hormones – cortisol and adrenaline - that increase your blood pressure and can also increase your likelihood of developing a clot in your arteries.

Stress can increase the production of these hormones which prepare the body to react to a new challenge. You may have heard reference to the 'flight or fight' response of the body, and this is in essence what your body is preparing for. Over the centuries, if you were facing a dangerous or challenging situation such as being confronted by a bear or going into battle (or a hoodie with a knife!) this was a very useful response as it diverted blood to the areas of the body that you would need to 'fight or run for it (flight)' but in our modern westernised society you have different challenges to face, which are not necessarily immediate or obviously 'dangerous'. If you are under pressure or feel stressed at work for a prolonged period of time, it can have a negative effect on your blood pressure.

Stress can also affect your state of mind and make you rely on quick fixes, rather than taking long term action to deal with the stress and prevent it building up. This can take the form of encouraging less healthy behaviours such as:

- over-eating
- smoking
- drinking too much alcohol
- taking recreational drugs.

You may also not sleep well at night which will also affect your state of mind too, and you may start to wake up early in an anxious state and not be able to get back to sleep. This can also mean that it discourages you from spending time on healthy behaviours such as physical activity or relaxation time.

It is important to identify the things that cause you stress, recognise when they might be affecting your health, and take action to reduce or avoid the stress so it does not affect your health.

One of the key factors that research has shown is that people are more likely to feel stressed if they feel that they have little or no control over their work, but have a lot of demands and targets placed on them to achieve. Research has also shown that people in manual jobs are more likely to be in stressful situations at work. Therefore the more you can do to control your work environment and objectives the more likely you are to have less stress. If you are able to take more control over this and influence your work targets and objectives the less likely you are to work in a stressed state of mind.

If I get high blood pressure can it be treated?

The good news is that high blood pressure can be treated. Once you have high blood pressure it is not generally something that can be cured, but it can be treated effectively, especially if you take steps to reduce your blood pressure yourself by adopting a healthy lifestyle. A lot of research has been done on how to treat high blood pressure effectively and there is now very good evidence about which drugs or medicines are the most effective, even if you sometimes need to take more than one medicine to keep your blood pressure under control. Research has also shown that lowering your blood pressure to normal levels reduces your risk or likelihood of having strokes, heart attacks, heart failure and kidney disease than may otherwise happen, as discussed earlier in this book.

Can my GP help me manage my high blood pressure?

In the UK you are most likely to have your high blood pressure treated at your GP practice or surgery, either by your doctor or by the practice nurse. In many surgeries nowadays you will more than likely be invited to come to a specific clinic at the practice where they will monitor your blood pressure (amongst other things), and make sure you are on the right drugs, or medication. Often as not these specific high blood pressure clinics are run by nurses, although they may also be run by or as well as pharmacists who are becoming increasingly involved in monitoring and managing this condition.

Sometimes it may be necessary for your GP to refer you to someone who specialises in managing high blood pressure. If this happens to you, you will probably be sent a letter giving you an appointment at the hospital, which is often where these specialists work. If you are referred to a specialist it is likely to be because your GP and/or practice nurse are having some difficulty in getting your blood pressure under control, and you may therefore have quite high blood pressure, or else be experiencing quite a lot of side effects from the medication (drugs) you are taking to control your blood pressure.

To see who else might be involved in your treatment see page 52.

So what does having an increased risk of cardiovascular disease actually mean?

The term 'cardiovascular risk' simply means determining what your personal risk of developing heart disease or stroke is. Your risk *can* be assessed by looking at several specific risk factors for heart disease and stroke. A risk factor is something which increases your likelihood of getting the disease.

The main risk factors for heart disease and stroke are:

⇨ High blood pressure

⇨ High cholesterol

⇨ Smoking

⇨ Not doing enough exercise/physical activity

⇨ Being overweight or obese

⇨ Having diabetes

⇨ Having a family history of heart disease or stroke

Your level of risk is calculated using certain information and measurements which are specific to you, such as:

• age

• gender

• blood pressure reading

• the cholesterol levels in your blood

• are you diabetic?

• do you smoke?

• ethnicity

The results of the calculation are then given to you in percentage terms of your likelihood of developing heart or stroke disease within the next 10 years. For example you may be told that you have a 9% chance of developing heart or stroke disease within the next 10 years. This means your risk is low to moderate. If you have a score of 20% or greater it means you have a high risk of developing heart disease or having a stroke within the next 10 years, and your GP will discuss with you what medication he would like you to take (see medication on page 39). However *there are several things you can do yourself* that will help to reduce your level of risk. The different risk factors that were identified when you had your risk score calculated will give an indication of which parts of your day to day lifestyle you would gain the most from improving. This could include eating a lower fat healthier diet, drinking less, taking more exercise and stopping smoking. If you change any of these things it is often known as adopting a healthier lifestyle, and literally means modifying your risk factors to improve your health.

Treatment Threshold if non-diabetic and no Heart Disease identified by doing a Cardiovascular Risk Score	
Low	0 – 10 %
Increased Risk	10 – 20 %
High	20 % or above

How often should I have my blood pressure checked?

One of the key aspects to maintaining your health is to have regular checks. Everyone should 'Know their Number' and know what their latest blood pressure reading is and be able to keep track of it and whether it is staying steady or varying.

Primarily you need to have your blood pressure checked at least every 5 years but it is a good idea to have it taken more often than this as you get older, so pragmatically every two or three years.

This is more relevant as you get older because your blood pressure will increase slightly with age. The only way of telling if it is going up is to have it taken regularly. If it is on the high side of 'normal', so between 130/85 and 139/89 mmHg, or if you have had a high previous reading in the past, you should ideally get it checked every year. If it is within the 'borderline' range (140/90 to 159/99 mmHg) it is very important to make any lifestyle changes that you can to lower it – see page 62. By keeping track if it is rising or not you can make changes to your lifestyle to help lower it.

Adopting a healthier lifestyle will help you keep your blood pressure within normal limits as much as possible. Obviously if you are seeing your GP or practice nurse more regularly about something else it is easy to ask to have your blood pressure checked while you are there, so that you can make sure you *Know Your Numbers* and have the most recent ones available. There is a chart at the back of the book to help you to keep track of your numbers.

When you make the appointment with your practice to have your blood pressure checked it would be a good idea to ask the practice to book you for an 'MOT' or health check. The most recent Department of Health policy – Putting Prevention First - has been set out to ensure that regular vascular or *heart health-checks* are done on everyone over the age of 40 years, so why not take the opportunity and be prompt in ensuring that you have your check sooner rather than later?

GPs and practice teams will be expected to routinely do these checks on people registered with them to make sure people who have a higher risk are identified. Those who have been identified as 'high risk' will be given medication, such as statins to lower your cholesterol level, aspirin and blood pressure lowering drugs if appropriate, and they will be closely monitored and worked with to help reduce their level of risk.

If you take responsibility and control and initiate the check, the earlier you will know if there is something that needs to be addressed with regards to your health. And remember that the sooner you make any lifestyle changes and reduce not only your blood pressure (if it is a bit high) but other risk factors for cardiovascular disease, the more likely you are to avoid or reduce the need for having to take any medication or suffering from long-term complications.

In order for your GP or practice nurse to make a diagnosis of high blood pressure you will need to attend the surgery several times to have your blood pressure taken. The reason for this is that if you have a one-off reading that is higher than normal it could be due to several things. For example if you have been rushing around just before you came to the surgery and you have not had long enough to sit and relax before the blood pressure was taken it could well be higher than usual. Another example is if you had been 'out on the town' the night before and had quite a lot of alcohol to drink this could also affect your blood pressure.

Since you are at your doctor's surgery it would also be a very good idea to get a cardiovascular risk assessment done at the same time so that you can take stock of how your overall health is, apart from your blood pressure.

> If you experience symptoms such as frequent nose bleeds or dizziness you should make an appointment with your doctor to check you over and find out what is causing your symptoms.

What tests am I likely to have?

The tests that you are likely to have done, apart from having your blood pressure measured, are urine tests, blood tests and an ECG or electrocardiogram.

The urine test is to make sure that your kidneys are working well, and especially that there is no protein in your urine, which could be an indication that the kidneys are not working at their best.

The blood tests are measured from a blood sample, and are routine to make sure that your general health is good. In particular your kidney function is checked to make sure your kidneys are working well (renal function test) and there are no signs of any damage. Your cholesterol will probably be checked as well.

The ECG is a test to show how well your heart is working. It does not take long to do and a machine is used to do it. Some sticky pads, or electrodes, are put on your skin in specific places to record the electrical activity of your heart. The printout gives a picture of how your heart is working. You do not feel anything during this test.

Your GP or practice nurse will explain your test results to you, and also explain how some of the tests will be used as part of an assessment to work out your cardiovascular risk score, or how likely you are to develop heart disease or stroke over the coming years. If you are unsure, just ask, as the nurses and GPs are there to help you understand about anything your assessment shows and what treatments are available.

Blood pressure measurement

Your blood pressure is taken using a machine or device called a sphygmomanometer, and will either be taken using an electronic machine or by the doctor or nurse using what is know as a 'manual device' and then listening for sounds with a stethoscope placed on your arm to hear what your blood pressure is. The newer, and now more common, devices are electronic machines where a cuff is placed on your arm and the machine is started off and then gives a readout of your blood pressure. Blood pressure is measured in millimetres of mercury – mmHg.

When the reading is written down you will see two numbers, like a fraction, such as 140/85 mmHg. The person taking it will tell you that it is 140 over 85. The top number records what the pressure is in your arteries when the heart is pumping blood out of your heart under pressure, and you may hear it being called the systolic. The bottom number shows the pressure in your arteries when your heart is relaxing between beats and it is filling up with the next lot of blood to pump out. You may also hear this number called the diastolic.

Your blood pressure may vary quite a lot during the day depending on what you are doing. It is generally lowest when you are fast asleep at night, or if you relax and do nothing. If you stand up or when you take exercise or feel very anxious your blood pressure will go up. This is normal. When you have your blood pressure taken it is very important that you are as relaxed as possible so that the doctor or nurse can get the most accurate reading of your blood pressure, so they will always take it after you have been sitting down for a few minutes, and preferably longer. That way you are very unlikely to have high blood pressure diagnosed incorrectly.

Sometimes your GP may decide that he/she would prefer to do readings at regular intervals over 24 hours. If this is the case they will ask you to come during the day and attach a small machine that is preset to take your blood pressure at regular intervals throughout the day and night. They will then ask you to keep it on your arm and come back in 24 hours time when they will take it off you and analyse the readings. They may do this if they feel that your blood pressure goes up when you come in for readings in the surgery, or just to get a better picture of how your blood pressure changes between day and night time.

What treatment can I expect for my high blood pressure?

First and foremost treating your high blood pressure will depend very much on two things:

- how high it is

- what other risk factors for heart and stroke (cardiovascular disease) you have

If your blood pressure is slightly raised i.e. between 140/90 – 160/100 mmHg you are very likely to be asked to make the most appropriate lifestyle changes specific to your health. Provided that you make these lifestyle changes successfully within a few months you will probably not need to take any medication (tablets).

However, for some people, whose risk assessment identifies them as being at high risk of developing cardiovascular disease over the next 10 years, they may be asked to take tablets as well, especially if they are a bit older or have other risk factors (described previously) for heart disease and stroke. These other risk factors will include a high cholesterol, if you smoke, or if you already have complications such as a previous heart attack or stroke.

The single biggest thing that YOU can do to keep your blood pressure within normal limits, especially if you have had one or two blood pressure readings which are raised but you have not had a diagnosis made yet, is to review and make positive lifestyle changes. These are discussed in more detail in the next chapter, but the key changes to make are:

- **Cut down** on the amount of **salt** you eat every day to 6 grams or less

- Eat at least '**5 a day**' - five portions of **fruit and vegetables** every day, and more portions if you are able to. The evidence is that eating 8 portions a day is even better for you, both in terms of heart disease and stroke, but also for bowel cancer etc.

- **Cut down** on the amount of **alcohol** you drink

- **Increase** the amount of **physical activity**, or exercise, you are doing. You should aim for 30 minutes at least 5 times a week to improve the fitness of your heart.

- **Lose weight** if you are overweight – if you are not sure what your ideal weight should be discuss it with your practice nurse who will advise you. They may also be able to refer you to weight management classes, stopping smoking support, and healthy eating advice and support, if they are unable to do it directly for you themself.

- **Give up smoking** if you are a smoker. See page 117.

What medication or medicines will my doctor put me on?

Your doctor will choose which tablet/s to put you on, as different medications work better in certain people, and you may need to take more than one type of drug to lower your blood pressure. If you and your GP decide that tablets, as well as making lifestyle changes, are the right treatment for you, then your GP will need to consider certain things about you. This will include if you have any other health problems, what your ethnic group is, and also how old you are.

If you are 55 years of age or older, or if you are of black African or Caribbean descent (although not mixed race), then the first choice for your treatment should be a drug called a calcium-channel blocker, or a thiazide diuretic. Diuretic drugs are also known as 'water tablets'.

If you are younger than 55 years, and not black, the first choice of treatment is likely to be a drug called an *ACE Inhibitor.*

ACE Inhibitors (ACE or ACE-I)

ACE stands for angiotensin-converting enzyme, and is one of the enzymes involved in the maintenance of your blood pressure. Some people develop a persistent cough when they are taking ACE inhibitors, which can be quite irritating. This is the most common side effect and if this happens to you, you should inform your GP or Practice Nurse, as you could then be offered a slightly different type of medication known as an *angiotensin-receptor blocker* (ARB) instead.

Drug treatment should be offered to patients if they have the following:

⇨ Consistently raised blood pressure of 160/100 mmHg or more

⇨ Blood pressure consistently above 140/90 mmHg and who have a raised cardiovascular risk of heart disease or stroke of 20% or more over the next 10 years

⇨ Consistently raised blood pressure above 140/90 mmHG and already have cardiovascular disease or have damage to their kidney function.

Many people need to take more than one type of medication to lower their blood pressure to a normal level. The 'NICE' guidelines, issued by the National Institute for Health and Clinical Excellence (see the 'Useful websites' section on page 121) make recommendations about which medications you should be offered and whether you need one medication or more. The aim of the treatment is to lower your blood pressure to less than 140/90 mmHg. This will be done as a combination of making lifestyle changes, adding drugs as needed, until your blood pressure is lowered to normal levels. Before adding in another medication to your treatment, your GP should make sure that you are on the right dosage for the drug you are already on. Obviously he or she will take account of any side effects or any other medical reasons that you may have for not taking the drugs.

It is really important to take your medication as directed so the GP or nurse can see how well it is working. If you experience any side effects you should inform your GP or nurse as soon as possible so that they can make any necessary changes in your treatment. Whatever you do - don't just stop taking the tablets. Under certain circumstances, for example if you are out of work and claiming benefits, you may be eligible for free prescriptions, so do check with your GP or Practice Nurse if you think you may be eligible. You can also pay reduced charges if you have several regular medications, so once again do check with your GP, or with the dispensing pharmacist at the chemist.

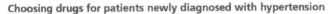

Choosing drugs for patients newly diagnosed with hypertension

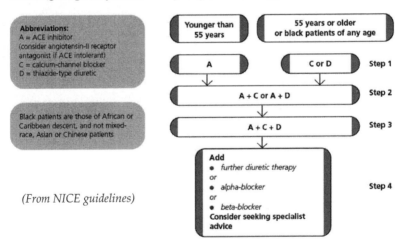

(From NICE guidelines)

Renin Inhibitors

This is a new group of drugs that work in a not dissimilar fashion to ACE-Inhibitors. They block renin production directly, renin being an enzyme that plays a major role in the body's mechanism responsible for maintaining blood pressure.

Thiazide diuretics

These are also known as 'water tablets or pills' and may be the first choice of treatment if you are 55 years or older, or if you are of black African or Caribbean descent (but not mixed race).

Calcium channel blockers

This is another class of drug that is an alternative to a thiazide diuretic if you fulfil the same criteria. These can have some side effects, including swelling of the ankles.

Beta-blockers

This is a class, or group, of drugs that were previously used as part of the management of high blood pressure but more recent research has proven them to be less effective than was previously thought. Their use nowadays, therefore, is much less common and is targeted at specific individual circumstances. However you may be put on them for other conditions, such as heart disease.

There are some other classes or groups of drugs that may also be used for managing high blood pressure, for instance *direct renin inhibitors*. However these other classes of drugs are not in common usage and will be prescribed for individuals by specialist doctors if they think they will be more effective in your specific circumstances. If this happens to you, you should ask your specialist to give you the information you need relevant to the specific drug.

If you are identified as being at high risk (a 20% or greater likelihood of developing a heart attack or stroke in the next ten years) you may also be started on a class of drug called a *statin,* to lower your blood cholesterol, and *aspirin* to prevent heart attacks.

See the 'Useful websites' section on page 161.

Effective Treatment needs to start early

We know that effective and early treatment of high blood pressure has a very big impact on the subsequent course of the disease by improving quality of life and reducing the likelihood of any cardiovascular events, such as a heart attack or stroke, or organ damage, such as to the kidneys. However, to be effective, treatment should begin within 3 months of having three or more readings of a raised blood pressure (between 140/85 and 160/95), and if making the necessary lifestyle changes has not brought it down to below 140/85. Treatment should also be started if your level of cardiovascular risk indicates that you have a greater than 20% likelihood of having a heart attack, stroke or related problem over the next ten years. Treatment needs to be effective to lower your blood pressure to normal levels. We know that drugs, together with leading a healthier lifestyle and making changes to improve your cardiovascular fitness, will seriously reduce your risk of having a future life-changing event and improve the quality of life.

Research is constantly producing new treatments to manage high blood pressure effectively. One of the latest research trials has shown that a combination of two drugs – amlodipine, which is a long-acting calcium channel blocker, and aliskiren which is a type of renin inhibitor – appears to have a better effect than single drug treatment or some other combined treatments. It is early days, however, to see if this is consistently effective and the final findings or results will be interesting to note. New research comes out all the time, and your GP should be up to date with the headline new treatments so you can always ask him/her.

Another way you can stay informed and find further information on the current treatments and new developments is by reading information on various useful websites such as the British Hypertension Society www.bhsoc.org, the Blood Pressure Association www.bpassoc.org.uk, and the National Institute for Health and Clinical Excellence www.nice.org.uk

Goals of therapy

- To lower your blood pressure to normal levels, and to reduce your risk of having a heart or stroke event in the next ten years

- Promote good general health and cardiovascular fitness

- Maintain a good quality of life

- Prevent any future cardiovascular events

Education and empowerment: This is the aim of this book - to teach you about your high blood pressure and put you in control of managing it. Information is power and gives you choices.

Practical self-management: Once you know how to manage your condition you can get on with living and make your diagnosis of hypertension, or high blood pressure, part of your life rather than letting it take over. Look out for the tips and hints throughout this book and check the websites listed.

Multi-professional team care: These are the professionals and specialists you can access to advise you on what to do and who can help you manage your high blood pressure:

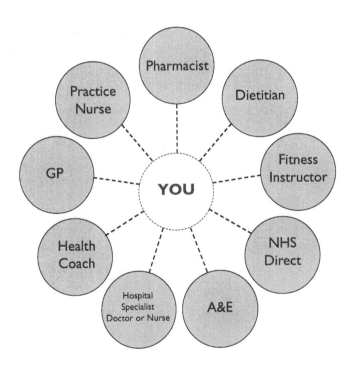

Meet the Specialists

I have recommended that you seek the help of various specialists in the diagram above. It is unlikely that you will need the services of all these professionals all of the time, but it doesn't hurt to know who they are.

Your GP

Your doctor is the first place to start as he can check your blood pressure and prescribe you the appropriate medication and send you for any further tests you may require.

Practice Nurse/Nurse Practitioner

Most doctors' surgeries have a practice nurse who will be able to monitor your blood pressure and answer any questions that may be concerning you about your condition and how you can make the changes needed to improve your health.

The Pharmacist

Your high street pharmacist is the best person to advise you on which medications can help you without a prescription. Use the same pharmacist for all your prescription and non prescription drugs as they can then monitor what you take and if there may be any unwanted interactions between different drugs.

The Dietitian

Most people would benefit from dietary advice. Simple advice can have a major impact on your weight and subsequently your general health and cardiovascular fitness. Unless you have other problems with your health or specific dietary requirements, following general healthy eating advice, especially in relation to your salt and alcohol intake, and eating a balanced diet as discussed in this book should suffice. The practice nurse at the surgery where you are registered will also be able to help you with this, and support you to make any lifestyle changes that are appropriate to your individual need.

The Fitness Instructor

Getting to know the fitness instructors in your local gym or leisure centre could be very valuable to you. Ask your GP to refer you to them especially if there is an 'Exercise on Prescription' scheme running locally as there will be some instructors trained up further with a more specialist knowledge of high blood pressure and cardiovascular disease. They can make sure that you have a programme that is suited to your specific needs and preferences and they will monitor your fitness levels both in general terms and also in relation to your cardiovascular health.

The Health Coach

People (are) wanting a different approach and services, looking for real choices, more local care, taking greater control over their health, support to remain independent...

Health coaching can form a vital part of support for someone with a long term condition (LTC) such as high blood pressure. It can best be described as 'the practice of health education and health promotion within a coaching context, to enhance the wellbeing of individuals and to facilitate the achievement of your health related goals'.

Health coaching can also be described as 'supporting you and your needs to become more active and self-reliant in your care.'

Similar to health education specialists, the coach usually takes an active and directive role, the coach helps you to achieve your goals by facilitating your learning process.

Coaching is a method of enquiring and questioning that helps you gain a better perspective and clarity. It brings structure and accountability that helps *you* focus more effectively on your health and lifestyle goals. You are naturally creative and resourceful and the coach's job is to provide support to enhance the skills, resources, creativity and strengths that you already have. While the coach provides feedback and an objective perspective, you are responsible for taking the steps to produce the results you want.

Increasingly people find using a health coach very beneficial as it helps you get your chronic condition in perspective. Coaches can help you to prioritise what is really important to you in terms of your health and the balance with the rest of their life.

Many people with LTC or life-changing medical/physical events get frustrated because they feel that their condition manages them and consumes their everyday life. Does this sound familiar?? Health coaching supports you to take control of your condition and manage it to become part of your every day life rather than the other way round.

Better and higher goals are set – ones that naturally pull you towards your health and life goals, rather than goals that require excess energy and resources to achieve. These skills translate into more success, and *you will* discover an amazing increase in what you can do if you have a coach.

If you want to find out more about health coaches you can always email me via my website and post me a question – **www.katygordon.com**. If you want to find a health coach local to you ask Google to do a search for health coaches in your area (**www.google.co.uk**).

The benefits of health coaching techniques are that it:

- Helps you clarify your vision and goals

- Enables you to set effective goals and priorities that honour your values

- Asks you to do more than you would achieve on your own

- Devises action plans with you to get results

- Guides you to create a more balanced and fulfilling life

- Keeps you focused on your vision of achieving bigger and faster results

- Provides the tools, encouragement, support and structure to accomplish more than ever.

NHS Direct

This is a useful service to offer advice if you are concerned and are unable to see your GP or practice nurse. They can help you make a decision on the most appropriate management and advise you who you should see for further advice. They also provide a lot of useful information on their website. Also see the Useful Resources section, **www.nhsdirect.nhs.uk**

A&E

Your local hospital A & E department is for accidents and emergencies only. It is there only if you think you may be suffering from a stroke, mini stroke or heart attack. Most chronic conditions are not an emergency and do not require the services at casualty. You will only have a very long wait as others are seen before you.

The more you know about your high blood pressure and of the drugs used to treat it the more able you are to then make choices and rational decisions about your treatment.

Remember, it is your life in your control! Have you identified any changes you need to make or learnt anything new from all this information that helps you make the most of your life for the future?

If you have, you might like to make note of it over the page so that you can make sure it is in your personal action plan.

Notes

Part 2

What you can do to help yourself

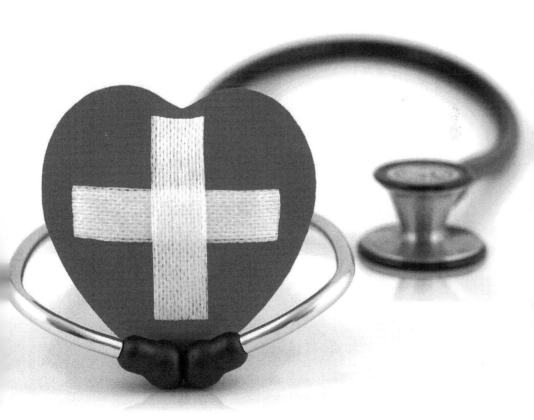

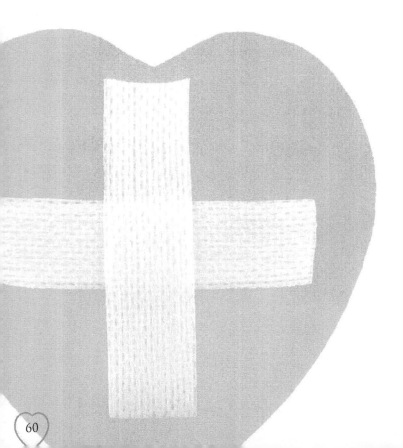

Where do I start?

There are two simple things which you can do to lower your blood pressure:

1. make changes to improve your lifestyle which will not only help to reduce your blood pressure but will also help to reduce your risk of developing any other related problems. This is often called self management.

2. make sure you take any medication or drugs that are prescribed for you as instructed by your doctor.

This section will help you think about your health and fitness in general, what you are currently doing that affects your high blood pressure and what you are doing to manage it. You should also consider who you can ask for advice. I have made a list of health care professionals and others on page 52 who may be able to offer you help to lower your blood pressure and keep self management as the key to controlling it and improving your fitness. As in all things only you, and you alone, know what is likely to work best for you in terms of how you approach things and who you might need to support you in making the healthy lifestyle changes you want to make.

Self Management

What can I do to lower my high blood pressure?

There are a number of things you can do to keep your blood pressure at a healthy level, and indeed lower or reduce your likelihood or risk of getting heart disease or of having a stroke in the future.

There are several key things that you can do to help keep your blood pressure down to a normal level, of which improving your diet and lifestyle are the most key things that you can do to make a positive impact on your health. These are also useful to follow if you have high blood pressure too.

- **First of all get your blood pressure checked regularly** (and your cholesterol levels too)

- **Eat less salt** – your salt intake should be no more than 6g each day – in real terms not more than 1 teaspoon of salt

- **Eat more fruit and vegetables** – eat at least your 5 portions a day. Each portion should be the size of the cupped palm of your hand.

- **Take regular exercise** – you should aim for 30 minutes of moderate exercise at least 5 times each week

- **Drink alcohol in moderation**

- **Drink at least 2 litres of water every day**

- **Keep your weight at a healthy level** – this means losing weight if you need to, and then maintaining your weight at this level

There are four other things you can also do which do not actively lower your blood pressure, but will improve your overall health and reduce your risk of having a heart attack, angina, a stroke or mini stroke in the future by reducing the risk of developing clots or narrowings in your arteries:

- **Stop smoking**
- **Eat a low fat diet but do not cut fat out altogether**
- **Manage and reduce your stress levels effectively**
- **Get a good night's sleep each night**

> **Reviewing and making positive lifestyle changes is essential but remember the key changes to make are:**
>
> - **Cut down** on the amount of **salt** you eat every day to 6 grams or less
>
> - Eat at least '**5 a day**' - five portions of fruit and vegetables every day, and more portions if you are able to. The evidence is that eating 8 portions a day is even better for you, both in terms of heart disease and stroke, but also for bowel cancer etc.
>
> - **Stop smoking** if you are a smoker
>
> - **Cut down** on the amount of alcohol you drink
>
> - **Drink** at least **2 litres of water every day**
>
> - **Increase** the amount of **physical activity**, or exercise, you are doing. You should aim for 30 minutes at least 5 times a week to improve the fitness of your heart.
>
> - **Lose weight** – if you are not sure what your ideal weight should be discuss it with your practice nurse who will advise you. She may also be able to refer you to weight management classes, stopping smoking support, and healthy eating advice and support, if she is unable to do it directly herself.

Some people like to monitor their own blood pressure at home. There are numerous devices or machines that you can buy, some taking the blood pressure from your wrist and others taking it from your upper arm, as is generally done in the doctor's surgery. My preference is definitely to buy one that takes it from your upper arm as it is much more likely that you will take a more accurate reading yourself using this type of machine. I have a machine made by Omron – the Omron M6 – but there are a lot of other machines on the market made by several different manufacturers. You should always do your own research as to what is right for you though. The Blood Pressure Association has a lot of useful information on its website if you are considering buying a machine to use at home yourself. The link to their home monitoring information is

http://www.bpassoc.org.uk/BloodPressureandyou/
Thebasics/Homemonitoring

It also has a very useful video to watch too. It is extremely important to make sure you buy a machine that has been clinically validated or in other words has been robustly tested and gives accurate results that can be trusted. You should also make sure that you buy the right sized cuff too – details of what you need to know are all included in the above link/website.

One word of caution: it is very easy to become a little obsessed about your readings so don't take them too often, and you should also take them at roughly the same time of day. There are various other things to be taken into consideration but rather than go into them in detail in this book I highly recommend that you visit the Blood Pressure Association's website and browse all the information there at your leisure.

Fitness levels

It is important not to overestimate your current level of fitness. Be honest with yourself and you will ensure that you start at the right place for you and see yourself progress quickly without any setbacks due to pain or illness. If you are an experienced exerciser looking at increasing the amount of training you are doing, it is just as important to be as realistic as a complete beginner. Even when you are feeling at your fittest be cautious not to do too much and pace yourself.

Remember, every little helps so use the stairs, walk to the next bus stop etc. If you are not very fit start small and build up. If you are in any doubt ask your GP or nurse for advice regarding the type of exercise most suited to you.

Weight

There is much evidence to say that losing weight will help lower your blood pressure. To know if you are over or under weight you will need to work out your BMI - or body mass index - first. (No, this BMI is not an airline!!) Your BMI is a measure of your body weight in relation to your height and is used to work out if someone is over or under weight. It is not flaw-proof as it does not distinguish between muscle and fat. (A muscular person may appear to be overweight when they are not.) Did you know that Cyril Smith (ex Member of Parliament) and Arnold Schwarzenegger had the same BMI? Which one do you think was overweight?

To work out your BMI look it up on the chart below.

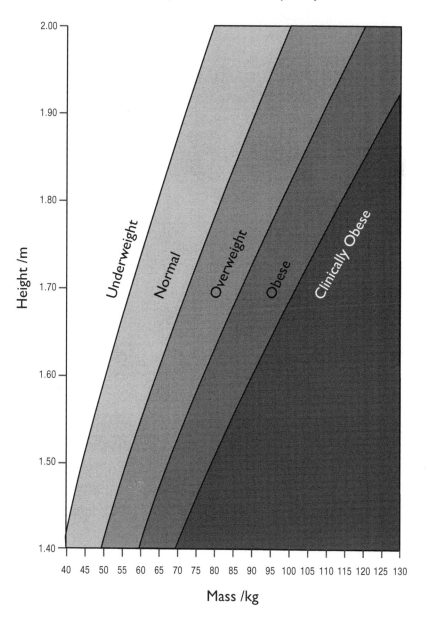

Body Mass Index (BMI)

The normal BMI range for men and women is between 18.5 - 24.9. If you have a BMI over 30, I would suggest you try to lose weight because your back and hip and knee joints will feel the benefits as you exercise if you are not as heavy. A healthy diet combined with a gentle walking programme is a good place to start and will prevent you putting too much strain on your body and prevent injury and illness. If you have any concerns you should have a chat with your doctor or practice nurse who can advise you and monitor you as you lose weight.

If your BMI is below 18.5 and you are in good health, don't worry. If you have lost weight recently without dieting or feel unwell you should see your doctor, you may need a review of your bloods or medication. *If you are a woman who has an irregular menstrual cycle or, regardless of sex, have issues with food, again you should see your doctor.*

For anyone who is not very fit and/or has not taken much regular exercise for quite a while I would also recommend enrolling at your local leisure centre and making an appointment with a fitness instructor who will devise a programme specifically for you and your particular needs. He or she will also monitor you on a regular basis to help you stay on track and encourage you. This also has the added benefit of making sure your programme is adapted to continue to be the best for you specifically as you get fitter. You will find some more information in the exercise section on page 103.

Healthy Eating

The information in this section gives you the basics about eating a balanced diet but if you want more detailed information I suggest you spend some time looking at the various websites and organisations listed on page 161, which will give the detail you are after.

Increasingly I think it is important to buy foods produced locally and in the right season – it reduces the carbon footprint and you will get the best nutritional value from them as they are fresh and have not been stored in chillers or part-frozen for 6 months. Plus you will also be supporting the local economy which has got to be a good thing. Personally I prefer buying from local farm shops, and I always get fish from my local market in Saffron Walden on a Saturday morning if I am home at the week-end.

Obviously, the cost of buying good quality food is prohibitive for many people – just try and buy the best quality you are able to afford.

Another thing to note is if you are buying frozen vegetables, check to see if they were frozen within 2 hours of picking – they will not have lost any of their nutritional value at all so you will get the maximum benefit from eating them.

I have tried to include things such as what a normal portion size is for each section. As a starter I recommend you go to the Food Standards Agency website, details of which are on page 162.

What is a healthy diet?

A good balanced diet is vital to provide energy and vitamins to keep our bodies healthy, grow healthy nails, keep our hair looking lustrous and our skin glowing. We need energy even when we are asleep to keep all our internal body systems working normally. We also need more energy when we are taking exercise. As our society has grown more mechanised our diet has not changed much to reflect the needs of our bodies. As a result there is a much higher level of overweight, obese and very obese people. What we should be aiming for is the amount of energy we eat or drink should equal the amount of energy we use every day. If this balances we will maintain our weight without too much thought.

However, we not only eat to feed our bodies with the energy we need, we also eat because we like food. If we continuously eat more calories than we use up we will steadily put on weight. Sadly the number of people in the UK who are overweight or obese is steadily increasing, but most worrying of all is the fact that more and more children and teenagers are getting obese. If you are obese you are at greater risk of having a high blood pressure, which is why it is important to lose weight if you need to and change your lifestyle to keep your weight at the right level for your height.

If you are overweight you should aim to lose a small amount every week and keep this up until you reach your target weight. Setting small, easier to reach goals each week will keep you motivated much longer than a huge goal that might easily appear impossible to achieve.

Many people think that the experts are always changing their minds because every few months the media publicises a story about some aspect or other of food which seems to be contradictory to previous messages. Often the scientific findings have been reported to the public before they have been fully researched leading people to think that once again the experts don't agree and that the message will change again in the near future. However the main messages about healthy eating have generally stayed the same for quite some years, if not decades.

I have based the information in this book on several sources. The advice taken from the Food Standards Agency UK website (www.food.gov.uk) provides consistent advice from their advisory authorities, and the guidelines they produce are consistent with well known research published in respected medical journals. They advise basing your meals on the "eat-well plate" which gives common sense guidance to food groups and how much can be consumed. It also categorises food into five major food groups, each of which should be eaten in the proportions outlined in the table below:

1.	Bread, rice, potatoes and other starchy foods	33%
2.	Fruit and vegetables	33%
3.	Milk and dairy foods	15%
4.	Non processed meat, fish, eggs, beans and other non diary sources of protein	12%
5.	Foods and drinks high in fat or sugar	8%

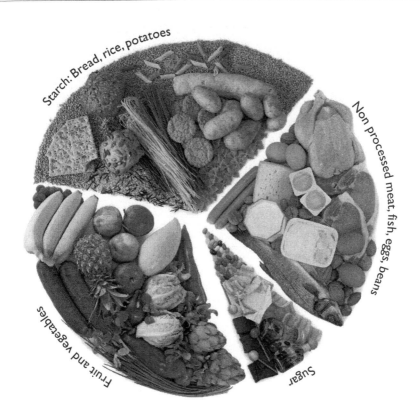

Always try to choose options that are lower in fat, salt and sugar when you can.

Food labelling

Under the Food Labelling Regulations of 1996 the following rules apply:

▶ Nutrition labelling is compulsory only when a nutrition claim is made, such as 'low fat'

▶ Labels need to give the amount of energy in kilojoules (kj) or kilocalories (kcal), protein, carbohydrate, and fat (expressed either as the amount of grams provided by 100gm or 100ml of the food)

- ▸ nutrient values can also be given per a quantified serving as well, but never instead of per 100gm

You can see from these regulations that not all food will have clear labelling advice which does not help when you are shopping in the supermarket and trying to make the right choices for your health.

Nutritional labelling on the front of the pack is designed to provide 'at a glance' information about the content of the pack. The Food Standards Agency recommend using a traffic light system where foods which provide a low proportion of your recommended daily intake of the main food groups (fat saturates, sugars, or salt) have a green label next to their respective nutrient, those with a moderate amount have a yellow label, and those with a high amount with a red label. However it is only a recommendation and some manufacturers have rejected the traffic light system and typically use Guideline Daily Amounts (GDA) which outline the number of calories, grams of sugars, grams of fat, grams of saturates, and grams of salt, and also give these figures as a percentage of the guideline daily amounts.

Until a single system is adopted and every manufacturer adheres to it trying to buy healthy options during your routine shopping remains something of a minefield, and somewhat off-putting for quite a few people, which is a huge shame. Eating healthily should be something that is easy to do, but as you become more familiar with the nutritional content of your favourite and staple foods it will become second nature if you persevere, and it is well worth doing.

Food groups, proportions/portions

There are several different food groups which make up our diets. One of the most important things to remember is that a balanced diet should contain all the food groups. Cutting right down on any of the food groups can be bad for your health because you could be missing out on vital nutrients. It is, however, important to get the right balance between the different food groups.

Carbohydrates

Starch is a really important part of a balanced diet. Starchy foods are a good source of energy and should make up approximately a third of the food we eat. Starchy foods are things such as pasta, rice, bread, potatoes and cereals. Most of us ought to be eating more starchy foods than we do, so think about the proportions of the different foods you eat each day, and if you are preparing a plate of food, once again, try to get the proportions in balance. It may take a little while for this to become a habit if you are not used to doing it but it will really help if you can change your eating habits to unconsciously incorporate this. Many of us eat less than we ought because we think that starchy foods are fattening, but in fact they contain less than half the calories you will find in fat. All you will need to do is to watch out for how you might use added fats in your cooking. By this I mean fat that you might use for things such as frying, or adding when you serve up a meal. It is this type of added fat which is where the extra calories are likely to pile on.

For those of you who are weight-watching, definitely try and eat the wholegrain varieties as they are a much better choice, although for healthy eating generally, we should all be thinking about this when preparing or eating a meal!

Reminder: It is always better to try and base your meals on starchy foods, rather than avoiding them, as they should make up around a third of your diet.

Starchy foods are also the main source of a variety of nutrients which are essential in a balanced diet. They also contain calcium, iron, fibre and the Vitamin B complexes.

Sugars are all too prevalent in our diets and definitely something that most of us should cut right down on. In the UK obesity is a growing problem (apologies for the pun!) and it has serious health implications. If you are overweight you have a greater risk of developing heart disease, stroke, and diabetes as well as high blood pressure. The more overweight or obese you are the greater the increase in risk so you can see how important it is to maintain a healthy weight.

It is all too easy to have too much sugar without even really thinking about it as sugar is present in many foods and drinks that we consume on a daily basis. There are the obvious ones such as cakes, sweets and biscuits, and fizzy drinks, but ice-cream, juice drinks and puddings are sometimes less obvious sources of high sugar content.

Whilst sugar occurs naturally in staple foods such as fruits and milk, which we don't need to cut down on, they are present in these other foods where sugar has been added and this is where we need to cut down on them or avoid them altogether. Apart from giving us unnecessary calories they can also cause your teeth to rot or decay. How many of us have been to the dentist to be faced with needing another filling? If we didn't consume so much sugary food the likelihood of this happening would reduce significantly.

Another point to note is that however much fruit juice (no added sugar) you drink each day the maximum amount it will count towards your 5-a-day is 1 portion...

Proteins

Proteins are an important part of our diets. We need protein to build and repair body tissue and they are also an important source of vitamins and minerals.

The main sources of protein are from fish, meat, eggs, pulses and dairy produce.

Fish is a good source of a whole range of essential minerals and vitamins. Breaking it down further, oily fish is particularly high in omega-3 fatty acids which helps prevent heart disease, and is also a good source of vitamins A and D. It should be noted that oily fish means fish such as mackerel, salmon, sardines, herring and trout and does not mean fish from your local fish and chip shop!

White fish includes fish like plaice, cod, haddock, monkfish and coley. They are very low in fat and are therefore a very good alternative to things like red meat which are higher in fat. They also contain some omega-3 fatty acids but not as much as the oily fish.

As part of our balanced diet we should be eating at least 2 portions of fish each week, and one of those should ideally be an oily fish.

If you want to make your diet even healthier you should think about how you cook your fish. Grilling, steaming or baking fish is far healthier than frying it, especially if it is deep-fried (as in the fish you get from your local fish and chip shop!).

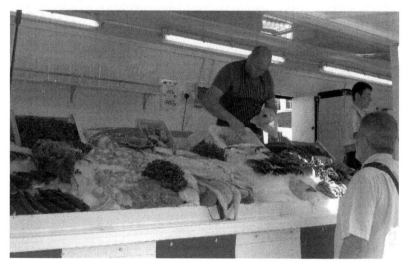

My local fish stall in the market. Crystal Waters Ltd, Lowestoft. See Useful Resources

Eggs are a good source of protein, as well as containing vitamins (A, D & B2) and minerals (iodine), and they are easy to cook. However you need to be aware to take extra care if you are cooking them for anyone who is vulnerable - the very young, pregnant, or elderly - as they can give you food poisoning if they are not stored and cooked properly.

There has been confusing information in the press about how many eggs you should, or should not, eat. There is actually no recommended limit on how many you should eat but it is useful to remember that you should eat a varied and balanced diet so having an egg-fest is not a particularly healthy idea!

Pulses (such as lentils, beans and peas), nuts and seeds are all another good source of protein and fibre, and also contain vitamins and minerals. Pulses also count as a portion of your 5-a-day, which is useful to know.

Pulses, in particular, are very versatile as they can be added to soups and casseroles as well as being served as a portion of vegetables in their own right. They can help supplement meat dishes as a form of protein too, which makes meals cheaper as well as being lower in fat, especially if you are on a low food budget. The fibre found in pulses can help lower your cholesterol, and also contains iron (although this type of iron is harder to absorb than that found in meat).

Nuts are an appetising food but are also high in fat so just remember to have them as part of a balanced diet. They also help protect against heart disease.

Meat is a good source of protein, minerals (iron, selenium and zinc) and vitamins (the vitamin B complex, and especially vitamin B12). However some types of meat are high in fat which can raise your cholesterol level, thus increasing your chance of developing heart disease. Eating leaner cuts of meat, and choosing how you cook it, such as roasting or grilling it, can make a big difference to eating more healthily.

As a rule the leaner cuts of meat are the most healthy options, and meats such as streaky bacon, sausages, beef burgers and pate are more likely to be much higher in fat content and therefore less healthy. Red meats are generally higher in fat than white meats, so chicken and turkey etc (without their skin) are better for you in general. Having said that venison and ostrich meat are two of the leanest red meats available. Meat products such as sausage rolls, pork pies, pasties etc are also much more likely to be high in fat, so eating less of these will help with your healthy diet.

Tips for cooking meat in a more healthy way

- Try using more pulses and vegetables in casseroles and then you can cut down on the amount of meat in the casserole

- Grilling meat is far healthier than frying it

- If you roast meat use a rack so the fat can run off

- Try not to add any extra fat or oil when cooking meat (a non-stick pan helps here)

- Eat more white meat than red meat

- Eat more portions of fish in a week which will also help cut down the amount of meat you eat

- Cut the fat off where possible and do not eat it

Dairy produce, such as milk, cheese, and yoghurt, are a very good source of protein, calcium, and vitamins A and B12. The calcium in them is easy to absorb and helps to keep our bones strong. However the fat content in these products can vary a lot and much of it is saturated fat which can raise the cholesterol level in your body which can then put you at increased risk of developing heart disease. There are various options open to you if you are trying to make healthier choices:

▶ Check the fat content of the cheese you buy most frequently and either buy reduced fat options, or

▶ Eat smaller portions, or

▶ Eat cheese less frequently

▶ Go for a lower fat milk, such as semi-skimmed, but remember, that fat contains important vitamins and minerals so you need to have some fat in order to get your fat-soluble vitamins

▶ Eat less cream and butter, or buy lower-fat options such as margarine

▶ Check the nutritional content of the labels on your favourite products so you can choose the ones that are healthier for you

Fats

Whilst a lot of people's perceptions are that fats are bad for you, it should be remembered that we *all* need to have some fat in our diets, not least because fat is a good source of energy, it provides essential fatty acids that the body can't make itself and also helps us absorb some types of vitamin. We perhaps just need to think carefully what type of fat and how much of it we eat, however, as eating too much of it can result in weight gain due to the high calorie content of fatty foods.

There are two types of fat found in food – saturated and unsaturated. If your diet is high in saturated fats then it can significantly raise your blood cholesterol level, thereby increasing your risk of developing heart disease or stroke. It is therefore very important to try to eat less fat overall, and to eat foods that are a good source of unsaturated rather than saturated fats.

So how can we do this? By eating less food that is high in saturated fat; by choosing options that are lower in saturated fat; and by choosing foods that have unsaturated fats rather than saturated.

It is important to try and remember which fatty foods are better for you to eat i.e. foods which are rich in unsaturated fats, and which foods you should eat less of because they are high in saturated fat. In the main, foods high in saturated fats include animal-derived foods: fatty cuts of meat, meat products such as pies, sausages, sausage rolls, salami etc; dairy products such as butter, lard, ghee, cream, sour cream and ice cream, cheeses (particularly the hard cheeses); cakes and biscuits; pastries; some sweet and some savoury snacks; chocolate; and coconut products such as coconut oil and cream, and palm oil.

Eating unsaturated instead of saturated fat can help lower your blood cholesterol level whilst also providing you with the essential fats that your body needs, and, as I have said earlier we need to eat some fat as part of a healthy balanced diet.

So what types of fat should we eat? Foods which are a rich source of unsaturated fats.

These are easier to remember as they are mainly contained in oily fish, avocadoes, nuts & seeds, and vegetable oils and spreads such as sunflower, olive, and rapeseed etc.

The following tables set out what you should eat more of and what you should eat less of:

Unsaturated fats	Saturated fats
Oily fish (e.g. salmon, trout, mackerel etc)	Fatty cuts of meat, sausages, pies, salami etc
Avocado/avocado oil	Dairy products such as butter, cream, crème fraiche, ice-cream, lard and ghee
Nuts and seeds	
Olive, sunflower, rapeseed and other vegetable oils	Cheeses, particularly hard cheeses such as cheddar etc
Spreads made from the oils above	Cakes, biscuits and pastries
	Some sweet snacks and chocolate
	Some savoury snacks
	Coconut oil and cream, and palm oil

Eat **more** of	Eat **less** of
At least 2 portions of oily fish each week – trout, tuna in spring water or vegetable oil	Red meat, hard cheese, salami, pate *NB fish & chips from the chippie don't count as oily fish!*
Eat sardines on toast as a light lunch or snack	Sausage rolls, meat pies, Cornish pasties
Low fat spread made from e.g. olive oil	Butter
Cook with olive oil, sunflower or rapeseed oil	Use butter, ghee, or lard sparingly or not at all
If you want a snack eat no more than a handful of unsalted nuts, or sunflower seeds or pine nuts etc *(Nuts are high in fat, so don't eat too many of them)*	Crisps and other snacks and nibbles as they can be high in saturated fats
If you are baking cakes use vegetable oil etc.	Don't use butter if baking cakes
If eating cheese, use lower fat options, and eat smaller portions of the softer cheeses	Cut down the amount of hard cheese such as cheddar you eat, and save it for a treat!

So what changes could you make to your diet that would be healthier with regard to fats?

You may hear people recommend diets such as the Mediterranean diet or the DASH diet. Both these diets are rich in vegetables, fruits, pulses etc and lower in meat and dairy products, sweets and sugar. The DASH diet is also lower in salt consumption, and the Mediterranean diet recommends moderate consumption of wine, and olive oil is a key component too. If you are interested in learning more about these diets you will find more information in the Useful resources section at the end of the book on page 161.

Vegetables and Fruit

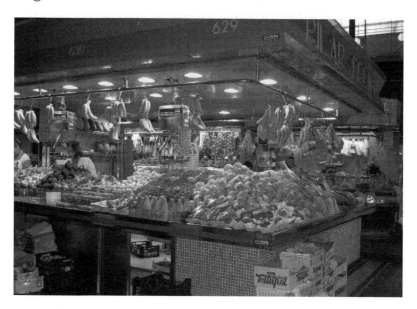

This is where we get most of our dietary fibre from each day. The main constituent of our dietary fibre is something called non-starch polysaccharides which come from plant cell walls. There are three types of these carbohydrates, but the main thing to remember is that they are not easily digested. This means that they will not stimulate much secretion of insulin which is necessary for regulating your blood sugar level, and is therefore very important in the management of diabetes. This also means that if you don't have diabetes and are generally healthy but you want to maintain a healthy weight these are good foods for you to eat.

Foods rich in fibre include vegetables, fruits, cereals, grains, pulses and wholegrain bread.

Diets high in fibre are associated with a reduced risk of:
► colorectal cancer (bowel cancer)
► heart disease
► stroke
► hypertension (high blood pressure)
► diabetes
► obesity
► gastrointestinal diseases (for instance, reflux, ulcers etc.)

They are therefore an important component of our diets.

Eating the recommended amount of dietary fibre helps:
► lower blood pressure
► lower the amount of cholesterol in your blood
► improves insulin sensitivity (in both diabetic and non-diabetic people)
► increase weight loss in obese people
► gastrointestinal function thus preventing the likelihood of developing things such as reflux, stomach and duodenal ulcers, diverticulitis and constipation

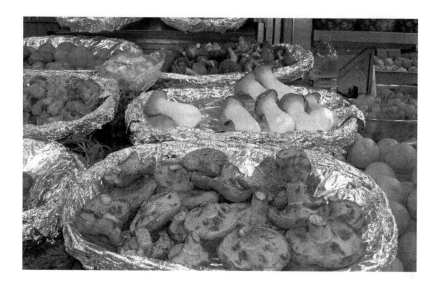

So, do you know what the recommended daily amount of fibre is? Many people don't but as I have said already, it is an important part of your diet. We should all eat at *least 5 portions* every day of fruit and vegetables. You can choose what form to eat them in, which gives you more variety to choose from: fresh, tinned, frozen, dried or as a juice. You should note though that you can't have all your portions as a juice. Only one portion a day of juice will count towards your 5-a-day. The other thing to note is that potatoes don't count towards your 5-a-day but they are important to eat as they are a starchy food.

So, the big question is: what is a portion?

ONE portion = 80g = any of the following:

- ▶ 1 apple pear, orange, banana or other similar size fruit

- ▶ 2 plums or similar size fruit

- ▶ ½ a grapefruit or avocado

- ► 1 slice of large fruit e.g. pineapple or melon

- ► 3 heaped tablespoons of vegetables, whether they be raw, frozen, tinned or cooked

- ► 3 heaped tablespoons of beans or pulses (however much you eat of these beans & pulses count as a maximum of one portion per day)

- ► 3 heaped tablespoons of fruit salad (fresh or tinned) or stewed fruit

- ► 1 heaped teaspoon of dried fruit e.g. mango, apricots, raisins, prunes

- ► 1 handful of cherries, grapes, or berries

- ► A dessert bowl of salad

- ► 1 glass of fruit juice (150ml) – as said earlier, however much you drink of fruit juice it will only count a maximum of one portion per day! Therefore drinking lots of smoothies every day doesn't count, unfortunately for those of you who think that it does!

You should also note that if you are buying fruit juices you should check for their sugar content. Some brands contain added sugar, and some contain very little fruit. Make sure you are buying brands which contain 100% fruit juice, and no added sugar. I used to buy fresh orange and raspberry juice until I realised that the producer of it added a very hefty amount of sugar – and I thought it was healthy!!

What effect does salt have on my body?

Although people have added salt to their food for centuries it is only in more recent modern times that this practice has become widespread. In Western countries the practice of adding salt is found everywhere, and salt can be added at any stage before, during and after cooking food. Not only this but salt is frequently added at any stage during processing of foods such as tinned foods, processed meats such as ham, bacon, smoked fish, soups, ready meals, some cheese and soft drinks etc. For some people salt is often added at all stages of cooking, resulting in wholly excessive use of salt on a daily basis, well over and above what we actually require to maintain a healthy body.

It has been estimated that of the amount of salt we eat every day 15% is added at the table or in cooking; 5% is naturally present in the food; and 80% is added by the food industry. Every day in the UK 26 million adults each too much salt! In the main this is because of the amount already in the food we buy from the food industry.

Salt has been known to be involved in high blood pressure since at least the 1960s but how salt leads to a chronically high blood pressure is not fully understood. Since the link is definitely there we should all be much more aware of how much salt we eat, whether it is in the obvious form, such as adding salt directly to our food, or in what is called 'hidden' salt. Hidden salt is more difficult to know about, because it is hidden in foods such as ready meals, tinned food, processed foods etc and is added by the food industry, so it is not easy to control.

Cutting down on salt reduces your blood pressure even if you don't have high blood pressure to start with. Since we already know that many people in the UK eat too much salt, cutting down the amount of salt you and your family eat anyway would be a good idea, regardless of whether any of you have high blood pressure or not, as the whole family would be much healthier and have a lower risk of heart disease or stroke at the same time.

There are two ways that our bodies maintain our internal salt balance: through our kidneys, in urine, and through our skin, in sweat. The main way of getting rid of excess salt is through our kidneys.

If our kidneys are working well, or normally, we can maintain the level of salt in our bodies on a daily intake of 1gram per day. Luckily our kidneys are wonderful organs which can regulate the right salt balance even if we eat much more salt than we really need. However, if we keep on eating too much salt, and our blood pressure stays higher than it should over a matter of months or years, eventually it will have a bad effect on our kidneys and they will start to not work as well. Taken to extreme, we can end up with kidney failure, and this is plainly something we want to avoid if we can.

Whilst we talk about how much salt we should eat per day we should actually view it as how much we eat as a quantity over a long period of time. What I mean by this is that even if our daily amount varies even by only a small amount, the quantity over time is quite substantial. Therefore if we reduce our salt intake and keep it much lower, day by day, month on month, it will have a significant impact over time on our blood pressure. This is very important for us generally, but particularly if our blood pressure is slightly raised, and even more especially if we know we have high blood pressure and are on treatment for it.

We know this because there are some groups such as Eskimos, northwest American Indians and the Masai of Africa who still live on a traditional diet (in other words the only salt they eat is what occurs naturally in their diet) and their maximum daily intakes are no more than 5 grams per day, and some of them eat less than 1 gram per day. High blood pressure is not common in these groups, and therefore we can assume that their diet plays an important part in maintaining a healthy or normal blood pressure, although there are other things which also contribute such as the amount of exercise they do.

Experiments have also been done on people who have normal blood pressures and who have been given additional salt to their diet in a controlled environment. This showed that they developed significantly higher blood pressure. In the face of all this evidence the obvious thing we all need to do is to significantly reduce or cut out adding salt to what we eat.

Let me tell you a story to illustrate this point.

A few years ago I was working closely with the Specialist Hypertension Nurse at the hospital I was working at. She had been referred someone who seemed to have completely intractable and dangerously high blood pressure. Over several visits this woman's drug therapy was changed in both what drugs she was prescribed but also in the dosage of them, and, amongst other things, she was also advised to not add any salt to her food at all. A few weeks later she came to see the nurse and said she had been watching a programme on television the night before and it had stressed the importance of not adding salt to anything because of the effect on your blood pressure. It had obviously raised a question for this woman which she asked the nurse: 'If I add salt to my coffee will that have the same effect on my blood pressure as adding it to my food?'

The nurse had previously asked her if she added salt to her food, and had advised her not to, but the woman had not thought drinks were included! They had a long conversation and it turned out that this woman added a teaspoon of salt to every cup of coffee she had because her grandmother had brought her up to do this. What's more she had several cups of coffee each day! Her grandmother had been brought up in the tropics and had been told by her family that she needed to add salt because of the amount of salt that was got rid of from the body by sweat which needed to be replaced. Hey presto! This was the main reason why this woman's blood pressure had been so high. She cut out the salt from her coffee (she had already stopped adding it to her food) and in a few weeks her blood pressure was within normal levels and she was on only a fraction of the drugs she had been taking to control it.

Unfortunately the amount of salt, over the years, had taken its toll and the woman's kidneys were not working quite as well as they should which meant that the hospital saw her regularly for check ups to keep an eye on the function of her kidneys. However, she still led a normal life, and at least any further damage to her kidneys had been reduced because of the changes she made in her salt intake.

It is thought that if we reduced the UK's average daily salt intake for adults to 6g we could prevent roughly 17,500 premature deaths each year. That is a staggering thought, isn't it! What effect would that have on the number of people who had high blood pressure? And even more thought-provoking, how many fewer people would have a stroke? How much salt could you cut down on, do you think?

So what does 6 grams per day mean in real terms?
As a nation we consume too much salt. According to NICE (the National Institute for Health and Clinical Excellence – see page 161) the daily recommended intake for an adult is no more than 6 g per day. In real terms this is about 1 teaspoon.

Most foods contain some salt, but it is the foods that are high in salt we need to be more aware of and avoid. Some foods are always high in salt because of the way they are made. If these are some of your favourite foods you can still enjoy them sometimes as a real treat but try and only have very small quantities of them. Over time if you can re-educate your taste buds to enjoy less salty foods you may even cut them out all together.

Using a salt substitute is not necessarily a good idea either as products such as Lo-Salt contain potassium. Too much potassium is not good for your health if used in moderate quantities, especially if you have heart problems. Too much potassium can lead to what is known as cardiac arrhythmias – irregular heart beats or rhythms, some of which can be life threatening.

Unfortunately the best thing to do regarding your salt intake is to bite the bullet and cut it down rather than use anything else. You don't want to run the risk of possibly having other health problems apart from your high blood pressure, do you?

In the following table a number of basic groceries have been taken from the website of a leading supermarket and the salt content of each food has been entered:

Food item	Mass of salt	%daily intake*
Hovis Granary Loaf – 1 slice	0.38 g	6%
30 g serving of cornflakes	0.7 g	11%
Own brand chicken curry ready meal	2.16 g	36%
Own brand Margherita Pizza	1.3 g	21.7%
Own brand British Breaded Ham – 1 slice	0.38 g	6.35
Own brand Salt & Vinegar crisps – 1 pack	1.11 g	18.5%
Own brand croissants – individual	0.4 g	6.6%
Heinz Minestrone Soup – ½ can	1.3 g	21.6%
Own brand pork sausage – single sausage	0.57 g	9.5%
Heinz Baked Beans – ½ can	0.6 g	10%
Potato salad – ¼ (small 300 g pot)	0.38 g	6.3%
Heinz Tomato Ketchup – 1 x 15 ml serving	0.2 g	3%

* assuming 6 grams, the recommended daily intake

From this one can see that it is very easy to exceed a 6 gram daily limit:

Breakfast:
- Cornflakes   (0.7 grams)
- 2 slices of toast   (0.76 grams)

Lunch
- ½ can Minestrone Soup   (1.3 grams)
- Ham sandwich   (0.38 + 0.76 grams)

Dinner
- Chicken curry ready meal   (2.16 grams)

Snack
- Salt and vinegar crisps   (1.11 grams)

This meal plan gives 7.55 g salt in one day. If we consider this only accounts for around 80% of the salt intake, the actual figure on this meal plan is closer to 9.4 g.

You will need to go and research what the salt content of your favourite foods are and see how high they are in salt. How about next time you are out shopping make time to compare the amount of salt in a few similar products, and then always choose the ones that are lower in salt? Small changes like this will make a big difference to your overall daily salt intake, which will also be much healthier for you.

The following table is taken from the Food Standards Agency website but gives you a good idea of the foods you need to cut right down on and only have as a treat every now and again:

Foods that are often high in salt

Try to eat smaller amounts of these, or have them less often.

- Anchovies
- Bacon
- Cheese
- Chips (if salt added)
- Gravy granules
- Ham
- Olives
- Pickles
- Prawns
- Salami
- Salted and dry roasted nuts
- Salt fish
- Smoked meat and fish
- Soy sauce
- Stock cubes
- Yeast extract

Foods where some brands/recipes are high in salt

Compare the labels on similar foods and choose the ones lower in salt.

- Bread products such as crumpets, bagels and ciabatta
- Pasta sauces
- Crisps
- Pizza
- Ready meals
- Soup
- Sandwiches
- Sausages
- Tomato ketchup, mayonnaise and other sauces

www.eatwell.gov.uk/healthydiet/fss/salt/whichfoodscont ainsalt/

As part of a healthy balanced diet you will not only need to work out what that means in terms of calories, proteins, fats and fibre and making sure you have a balanced plate, but also how you are doing on your salt intake too. If you are used to having quite a lot of salt in your food try substituting salt with herbs for flavour in your cooking. If you like strong flavours try using mustard oil instead of butter, especially when cooking Indian food. As your taste buds start to acclimatise to a less salty diet you may initially find that your food tastes blander but you will find that gradually you notice a much wider range of flavours and tastes in your food that you didn't taste before, and that you start to enjoy more subtle flavours.

Maintaining a healthy balanced diet is not necessarily that easy to manage if you haven't looked at all of these things before, is it?

How much water or fluid do I need to drink?

Much has been written about making sure you drink enough water but there has not been a lot of research done to back this up. The message that we should drink at least 8 glasses of water or about 1¼ litres each day is an important one to stop us from getting dehydrated. We obviously need more if we are in a hot climate, or during the summer.

In the days when I worked on general wards it was often the junior student nurses' job to make sure that all the patients had enough to drink during the day and for some patients, we used to have to write on a fluid chart each time we gave them a drink and how many millilitres each drink was. By doing this we could see if someone was falling behind with their fluid levels. This was especially important if they had a high temperature as they would lose more fluid because of it.

Water is essential because most of the chemical reactions in the cells in our bodies need water as part of the reaction. Water makes up ~80% of our bodies so you can see how important it is to make sure we drink enough water every day to maintain that balance. We also get some fluid from food we eat, as well as from what we drink. Remember that water is in other fluids we drink, although I think we are talking about non-alcoholic drinks in particular, as alcohol can cause dehydration!

We lose water from our bodies in a variety of ways, the most obvious being what we lose through our kidneys in urine. Urine also contains some of the toxins and waste products produced by/within our bodies. We also lose water when we sweat, through our lungs and respiratory passages when we breathe and we also lose some water through our faeces.

The amount of water we drink in and the amount of water we lose through urine and sweat etc should be balanced and under normal circumstances we should aim for about 2,300 mls per day. However, prolonged exercise can make this rise quite considerably and we can lose up to as much as 6,000 mls in a day. To stay healthy we must replace this in order to keep the right water balance in our bodies.

It is therefore a good idea if you are in a hot climate, as well as if you are doing strenuous exercise, to remember that you have increased water requirements and make sure you remember to drink more water.

It has been reported that drinking tea and coffee can cause you to pass more urine and can therefore dehydrate you. However, more recently some research has been done which says that this does not seem to be the case and that you can count tea and coffee as part of your daily fluid intake as well as water.

Does alcohol count as part of my daily fluid intake?

The same cannot be said of alcohol though! A small amount of alcohol may significantly reduce the risks of heart disease or stroke, and reports suggest that 1-2 units daily may reduce your likelihood of having a heart attack or dying. However, a long term excess of alcohol, and especially binge drinking, has been proved to greatly increase your risk of having a heart attack or stroke, and certainly increases your blood pressure. It is also associated with an increased risk of getting cancer, particularly mouth, oesophageal, liver and breast cancer.

In the UK the government "Drink Aware" guidelines reflect the evidence concerning the harmful effects of alcohol, and the range of about 2 units per day (light to moderate alcohol consumption) seems to have some positive health benefits. However you should have at least a couple of days each week where you do not drink alcohol, as apart from the effects on your blood pressure there are also effects on the liver, which excretes alcohol, and which needs to have some 'time off'.

So what does moderate alcohol consumption mean in practical terms?

The UK government guideline specifies that:

► 'A man should not regularly drink more than 3-5 alcohol units a day'
► 'A woman should not regularly exceed more than 2-3 units a day'

One alcohol unit is 10 ml or 8 grams of pure alcohol.

In practical terms the following table gives some guidelines to base your assessment of your alcohol intake on:

Drink	Number of units
Pint of Beer (5-6% alcohol)	3 units
A standard 175 ml glass of red wine (11-12%)	2 units
Small measure of spirits 25 ml (38-40%)	1 unit
Pint of strong cider (9%)	5.1 units

So a woman could have a glass of red wine at night, and perhaps a small measure of spirits. A man could have a pint of beer, and a glass of red wine. Any more than this is over the recommended limit. However, the alcoholic beverage industry does not make it easy to assess how much alcohol we have had. Some beers contain as much alcohol as the example of strong cider in the table above, and quite a few wines are 14-15% which is also more than the example given in the table above. Also quite a few wine bars, pubs etc offer wine in 250 ml glasses which will also dramatically increase the amount of alcohol you are drinking.

You can find more information about the alcohol guidelines on:

www.drinking.nhs.uk/questions/number -of-units/

www.drinkingaware.co.uk/

We can see that if you are not aware of what each type of alcohol means in terms of units/day that it is all too easy to drink excessively and risk negative effects on your health. Since excessive alcohol intake has quite an effect on our blood pressure it is all the more important that we know how much we are drinking and make sure we stay within the recommended limits as a general rule of thumb.

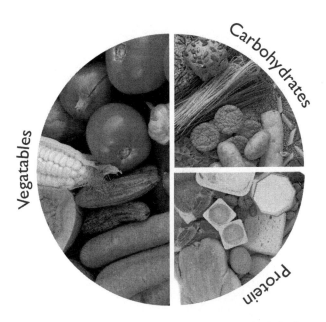

A balanced plate of food. Vegetables ½ of the plate, Carbohydrates ¼ of the plate and Protein ¼ of the plate.

Physical Activity or Exercising

We hear it everywhere – exercise is important, it helps keep you healthy. That's true for everyone. But what's less well known is that when people start exercising to lose weight, or just to get fitter, they find that a side effect of introducing exercise into their lifestyle is that they quickly reduce their blood pressure. This is especially so when it is used alongside some of the other changes we have discussed such as eating healthily, reducing the amount of salt you take in, cutting down on drinking alcohol and cutting out smoking.

There are three key elements to influence your choice of exercise. You might find it easier to think about it in terms of cost and how much you can afford to spend on exercising and improving your health generally. Plainly this is mainly dependent on your income and how much you can afford to budget for. Exercising at home will be the cheapest option although it has its drawbacks in that you will be exercising completely unsupervised. For those who might have more available income to spend on their health there are endless options. This could mean joining a gym, going to exercise classes at it, having an individual programme devised by one of the fitness instructors, right through to hiring a personal trainer and leaving them totally in charge of your fitness programme. Only you know how much you can afford to spend and what will work the best for you, in other words, what your motivation is like to get up and out there and start exercising.

Before you even think of starting to exercise you should do some research into what is available to you locally, how much it costs, and what your preferences are in terms both of cost and of what activity or activities you like to do, either indoors or outdoors.

> Appropriate exercise can have all sorts of beneficial effects, especially when used in conjunction with the right medication. Sometimes, in fact, in cases of mild hypertension, the right exercise may mean you don't need to take any drugs at all.

People's perception of exercise is often the gym, running etc. Gentle persistent exercise is great and need not cost anything. It is the small repeated changes that can make a difference especially if you are not very fit, rather than three times a week exhaustion in a gym. It's worth bearing in mind that a lot of housework is very good exercise!

> It goes without saying that if you feel sick, unwell, have pain or have a temperature you should stop exercising. If you get symptoms during or after exercising it is also important to see your GP for advice and just in case your medication may need to be changed.

So what questions are you likely to ask yourself about exercise, physical activity, moving your body more or whatever the word or phrase is that you use which means getting fitter…

Why is exercise so important for your body?
What does it do?

There are many reasons why keeping yourself physically fit is important. Not least is because it helps you maintain a healthy weight as part of a balanced lifestyle. It also keeps your heart and circulatory system healthy which very much reduces the risk of developing high blood pressure, heart disease and stroke. It keeps your muscles toned and fit which also helps keeps your bones healthy.

It's important to point out that although exercise will increase your blood pressure while you are exercising, it will however lower your blood pressure overall. It does this by a few different mechanisms, but mainly by helping your heart to be a more efficient pump.

If I am very unfit how much exercise or physical activity should I aim for?

If you are very unfit you should see your GP before you start to do anything. Your GP may be able to refer you to a local exercise on prescription scheme, if you have one in the area, which would be the best way of starting. Otherwise a fitness instructor at the leisure centre or a local gym would be the best person to assess you and devise a fitness plan that is right for *you*. The most important thing to remember is to start with small goals and then you are far more likely to achieve them. Beware - if you set yourself big goals it may be difficult to achieve them and you may become demoralised if you do not see much progress, which is not good for your motivation.

What/who else could help me?

Set yourself some simple, achievable goals at the start of your fitness plan which you could discuss and set with a professional such as your practice nurse, or a fitness instructor at the local leisure centre, or a personal trainer - whoever will be most helpful to *you* during the coming weeks and months to come as you get steadily fitter.

Keeping an activity diary and writing in it how much exercise you take each day (in minutes) and what type of exercise. Also using the modified Borg scale, discussed later in this section, while you are exercising and writing down each session what level you felt you were at for most of the time your were exercising. You could also write down the information you got from your heart rate monitor if you are a person that likes to use that kind of tool to help you. If you are working with a professional, which is what I would recommend, to monitor your progress and to provide support such as I have mentioned in the paragraph above they will find it very helpful to review your progress with you using the diary. If they have given you a personal regime to follow (fitness instructor or personal trainer) they will also be able to update it to make sure you are making the most of your fitness/activity sessions.

Even a friend or relative can be a good source of motivation and encouragement to help you keep up your exercise. You could even encourage them to exercise with you!

What resources are available to me to access as part of my fitness plan?

This depends very much on what types of activities you like to do. Apart from the obvious things like walking, cycling, swimming etc which you can do by yourself or with your family there are usually numerous groups or clubs you could join locally.

These could include:

▶ Leisure centres, both local authority and private gyms. The local authority-run centres may well have introductory schemes and also exercise on prescription schemes. Ask your practice nurse or GP if there are any special schemes running locally which could apply to you.

▶ Sports clubs, such as football, running, archery, canoeing, tennis.

▶ Walking groups – these are usually led by a trained walk leader and usually offer a selection of routes with different intensity, length and degree of difficulty so choose one that suits your level of fitness and you can progress through the different levels over time. The Ramblers Club (see the Useful Resources section at the end of this book) may also run walks in your local area, as also may Walking for Health (see page 163).

▶ Parks and Open Spaces – increasingly lots of parks are offering all kinds of facilities for all sorts of activities, from ball games of various sorts to open air fitness classes such as those run by British Military Fitness (see Useful Resources section at the end of this book), jogging and walking routes, skateboarding areas etc.

▶ Green exercise can include other sorts of outdoor activities such as gardening (your local authority might have some allotments available), nature conservation activities such as dry stone walling, hedge-laying and other such things. The National Trust (see Useful Resources section) runs carbon monoxidesome very interesting and different activity courses and holidays such as these, where you tend to meet like-minded people.

▶ Active Travel – many people walk, jog or cycle to work or the shops as a way of keeping fitter, as well as being greener and eco-friendly. You don't have to walk all the way but could get off the bus one or two stops early, or walk one way and get the bus back.

Your local Citizens Advice Bureau should have a list of what activities are available locally and their contact details so it is worth visiting them to find out what things you can do.

The Modified Borg Scale

	No.	Effort	Feelings/symptoms	
amber	0	Nothing at all		
	0.5	Just noticable		
	1	Very weak	Hardly any symptoms	
	2	Weak (light)	Aware you are moving, doing something	
green	3	Moderate	Fine, no problems	
	4	Somewhat strong/hard	Breathing a little stronger, able to talk when exercising	
	5	Strong/heavy	Feeling warm, a little out of breath	
	6		Feeling more out of breath, having difficulty when exercising	
red	7	Very strong	Perspiring	
		You should never exceed level 7		
	8			
	9			
	10	very, very strong/hard	Exhausted	

When exercising or walking, you need to be able to measure your exertion level or effort, without comparing yourself to others or thinking about the physical load. Ideally you should be exercising between levels 3 to 6 and you should *never exceed level 7.*

Guidance, support and advice

Before beginning your training programme it is important to be first seen by your GP or practice nurse. I also recommend, especially if you're new to exercise or have not trained for a long time, that you try and get the help of a personal trainer or instructor. I say this because it is almost impossible, in a book like this, to provide you with the exactly tailored set of exercises, with the right intensity and lasting the right length of time, to have the maximum beneficial effect for you. However, I know that personal trainers or instructors cost money, so you will obviously have to look at what options you can afford, and also what will work for you apart from the cost side of things. Even if you just see a trainer once, they can help you in setting the right goals for you and give you the information to assist you reaching your goals in the most efficient way. Another option is making an appointment with a fitness instructor at your local leisure centre, who can also supervise and monitor your progress.

When finding the right personal trainer for you, there are a few things to look out for. Firstly check that your trainer is insured. Ask to see their qualifications and even their testimonials. A good trainer will be used to this and will not mind at all. Whilst there are many qualifications that enable someone to call themselves a trainer look for ACSM (American College of Sports medicine), NASM (National Academy of Sports Medicine), NSCA (National Strength and Conditioning Association) and FASTER (www.fasterglobal.com).

This is by no means an exhaustive list but I would expect a trainer with experience in working with people who have been diagnosed with high blood pressure to have one or more of these qualifications. You could also use the national register of exercise professionals (www.exerciseregister.org) or national register of personal trainers (www.nrpt.co.uk).

Also check with your GP or local community leisure facility for ideas on new activities or classes to try. Many GPs will provide an 'exercise prescription' to refer you to a local programme.

A trainer or instructor may also have direct links with GP referral schemes and exercise on prescription programmes. This is a great place to start if you are unable to afford one-to-one trainer. Many local authorities run GP referral schemes through your local gym or leisure centre. It is well worth checking here first. Community leisure facilities are a super way to try new types of exercise as they tend to have a wide variety of activities in the one place and a full programme of classes to suit all levels.

What are the effects of exercise?

So how much change in blood pressure can you expect from your new exercise programme? As a guide the level of reduction in blood pressure from exercise may be in the region of 5–7 mm Hg after a single intensive exercise session or after a consistent series of regular exercises. In addition, blood pressure goes down for up to 22 hours after an endurance exercise session. It is worth noting that even very small changes in your blood pressure can have a massive effect in reducing the risk of stroke and coronary heart disease.

Directly after exercising, a drop in blood pressure is a natural and expected response. As muscle contractions help pump blood back to the heart, once you stop exercising and these contractions dissipate, the heart responds by decreasing cardiac output and so your blood pressure drops. A vigorous bout of exercise also dilates the blood vessels, which means less resistance to blood flow and a drop in blood pressure.

Make sure you know what happens to your normal heart rate during exercises of different intensities. Try using the modified Borg Scale and think about your whole body's response to the exercise you are doing. Ideally you should be exercising at the level of intensity that lies within levels 4 to 7 on the modified Borg Scale. You should not be exercising at all above level 7 unless you are with a fitness instructor, personal trainer, or have a very good level of fitness to start with and know a lot about the effects of exercise on your body.

Keep in mind that the aim of exercise is to create a more efficient system and by doing so place less strain on your heart and therefore lower blood pressure. It is important to measure exercise intensity so that progression can be planned at an appropriate rate and so that you can see your progress. Another way to measure your exercise intensity is by using METs or metabolic equivalents. You'll find these on most cardio machines in gyms.

Setting goals

A clear goal will help motivate you to start an exercise programme. Think of an event coming up in the near future such as having lunch with a friend or a holiday you have planned? Plan how you would like to feel on that day - how much weight have you lost? How much fitter do you feel? What are you wearing? What positive things do people say to you? Write these thoughts down in your action plan at the end of this book and plan your exercise to help you meet this goal. Make sure you keep your goals realistic. You know your body best and what you are capable of. When you've achieved it - celebrate! Why not then set a new goal?

Recommended programmes

For people with borderline or mild hypertension, the ACSM recommends following an exercise program that includes at least 30 minutes per session, most days of the week of moderate intensity. If you are new to exercise, I recommend you begin with 15 minutes and build up gradually.

Please note that if you have been recently diagnosed as having high blood pressure and you are now taking medication/drugs to control it you MUST check with your GP or practice nurse that your blood pressure is properly under control first. If it is still quite high you are at an increased risk of developing further problems.

I would recommend that you aim for moderate exercising when you first start. Your focus should be on incorporating this as part of a healthy balanced lifestyle, and not the sole focus.

People with hypertension whose blood pressure is not fully controlled, should not be doing vigorous exercise. Caution should also be taken with heat stress as some antihypertensive drugs can make it harder to regulate your body temperature. Other types of antihypertensive drugs can also slow your heart rate down which makes it difficult for your heart to pump enough blood round your body if you exercise vigorously. If you are on a beta-blocker you should ask your GP's advice as to what physical activities would be best for you to do, as beta-blockers prevent your heart rate from increasing too much depending on what dose you are on.

Proper breathing techniques should be followed and certainly you must not hold your breath as this increases thoracic pressure, which will push your blood pressure up and put strain on your heart.

If you are being supervised, or are having regular reviews by a fitness instructor they can keep you on track as to how much exercise you should be doing, and also by how much you should be increasing it provided you are not having any injuries or problems with your muscles etc.

Getting it right for you

The key thing to remember is - start at a pace that is manageable for you and increase frequency and intensity SLOWLY.

Once you've started - adapt your training slowly, only one variable at a time. For example, if you start walking for 20 minutes 2-3 times a week you could EITHER try extending this to 25 minutes 2-3 times a week OR walk for 20 minutes 3-4 times a week. Keep a diary of your exercise - you will be able to monitor your progress towards your goal and this is great for motivation. You can monitor your progress in the personal action plan at the end of this book.

Make sure you choose an exercise you enjoy. Moderate aerobic exercise (the rhythmical motion of your whole body), for example walking, is shown by research to be the most effective at lowering resting blood pressure. If walking is the exercise you choose, think about walking on a variety of surfaces - grass as well as pavements - this will be better for your joints. Think about your daily routine and where exercise might be able to slot in - you could even start with taking the stairs instead of the lift.

I believe there is an exercise/sport for everyone. There are so many choices and classes/groups to join. Have a look at community centres in your area, look on the web to find out groups for a new activity that you want to try. There are group dance classes for all levels, group walks, tennis, rowing, boxing (circuit training not sparring) exercise classes, cross-training and a whole variety of team sports. If you're not sure where to start try online facilities such as meet up group (www.meetup.com) or Facebook (www.facebook.com). It's a great idea to exercise with a friend - you can keep each other on track and you're much more likely to keep going if you have to match yourself with someone else.

There are also great options for exercising at home if you're into computer games. The Wii or Xbox have games that can get you up and moving. The Wii Fit has tools to assess your progress and basic fitness levels. There's a wide choice of games to suit all tastes and can be played by you or get the rest of the family involved.

Whatever exercise you choose it is important that you warm up and cool down correctly. Warm up with small, slower paced movements that reflect the activity you are about to do. This allows your muscles to start increasing their blood flow and get ready for the exercise you're about to undertake. Similarly, it's important to cool down after exercising and not stop suddenly. Cooling down helps your body and muscles to return to their resting state. If exercise is stopped suddenly the heart continues to pump additional blood around the body and you may feel faint as the blood isn't assisted in returning to the heart and lungs. Some antihypertensive drugs may cause blood pressure to drop too low if exercise is stopped abruptly.

What should I wear? - a note on kit

The most important thing is your shoes. Generally you will need trainers. If you're going to be walking or running, a good pair of running shoes is definitely worth investing in. Make sure you get a shoe suited to the type of exercise you plan to do - the key is to make sure your foot and ankle are well supported so you don't do any damage.

For the rest of your kit it really doesn't matter as long as you feel good and you're comfortable. In most sports shops you will find kit with technical fabrics that help to keep you cool whilst you train by wicking the sweat away from your skin. These are nice but not essential.

You know your body best and now you have information to make smart choices to improve your health so that you will enjoy a healthier future.

Stopping Smoking

Now then, for all you smokers out there it doesn't need me to tell you that it is not good for your health!!! Smoking is associated with so many diseases, both killer and causing long term disability, that if you haven't thought about giving up by now I would have to ask if you have a death wish???!! Do you seriously want to continue playing Russian roulette with your health?

Specialist Department of Health/NHS advice can be sought at www.smokefree.nhs.uk/ You can also find out on this site where and how to access your free NHS local service

On page 161 you can find a list of useful websites which can give you more help and information.

I am not going to go into all the whys and wherefores of giving up smoking because there is so much specialist help available on the NHS (access to this specialist help can be found through various organisations and agencies, a couple of which I have given above) but here are some facts that you might like to bear in mind:

Approximately 10 million adults smoke in the UK, which equates to roughly one sixth of the whole population. In percentage terms this means that approximately 22% of men and 21% of women are smokers. This is less than half the number of adults who smoked in 1974 and is obviously a good step in the right direction, but it has taken ~35 years to decrease the smoking rates by half. Unfortunately the effects of smoking can take a long time to manifest themselves. Conditions related more directly to smoking such as lung cancer, heart disease and stroke are well known in the UK but we are now seeing the numbers of people with chronic lung (respiratory) problems and conditions increasing, such as bronchitis and emphysema, and they will continue to increase for some while to come. Smoking can also affect your fertility and there are increasing numbers of couples who are turning to IVF in order to have a family. As it is, nowadays *in the UK it is recognised that tobacco consumption is the single biggest cause of preventable illness and early death.*

This obviously has a major impact on individuals and families health-wise, as well as an impact economically on their lives. This also impacts on the wider economy in terms of sick days paid for by businesses and employers, as well as nationally ensuring that the NHS can provide the right treatment for the related illnesses as early as possible, and in the event of that not being early enough, good hospice and care for people at the end of their lives.

Government expenditure in terms of education campaigns cost the nation £23.38 million in 2008-9, and cost a further £73.5 million on helping people to quit smoking. In the same year revenue raised for the government from tobacco taxes generated a massive £9.70 billion gross (£8.22 billion net of VAT).

Another interesting fact is that smoking rates are significantly higher amongst poorer people, despite the increasing cost of being a smoker.

A person who smokes 20/day will spend roughly £2000 each year on cigarettes, of which ~76% goes straight to the government in taxation. That is an incredible thought especially in times of an economic downturn – smokers, as a distinct group, are contributing, some would say well over the odds, towards government funding. Many would ask 'how do they afford it?'

In 2008 29% of people who worked in manual jobs smoked compared to just 14% of those in professional and managerial jobs. Again it seems incredible that the higher percentage of people who earn less in manual jobs somehow manage to actually afford it. Or is it that they are spending less on other areas of their life – compromising their lifestyle in order to smoke? If that is the case, what further detrimental effects will it be having on their health?

Can you really afford to smoke?

Passive or second-hand smoking also increases your risk of developing smoking-related illnesses or death, so if you are living with someone who smokes they are putting both of you at risk of developing smoking-related illnesses. If this is the case for you how much are you prepared to let the person you love jeopardise your good health or do you enjoy playing Russian roulette with it? What price do you put on having good health? What would it take to encourage them to stop smoking?

Children exposed to second-hand smoke are more likely to have ear and respiratory infections, and to die of cot death. Babies and children who grow up in a smoky atmosphere are twice as likely to have asthma and get chest infections, get ear infections and glue ear (which can lead to partial deafness), and are likely to be off sick from school more often.

A good friend of mine gave up smoking because she wanted to make sure that she was around to celebrate her daughter's 21st birthday (her daughter was ~4 years old at the time). She realised that if she didn't stop there was a significant chance that she might not be around, a price she wasn't prepared to pay. She also wasn't prepared to put her daughter's health at risk either through passive smoking.

Higher tobacco taxes reduce the amount of cigarettes smoked so the price of cigarettes has a major influence on cigarette consumption. However there are still a significant number of people who smoke living in the UK. According to surveys done, 2 out of 3 smokers would like to quit...

Deaths from smoking

Roughly 114,000 people who smoke in the UK die from smoking related illnesses each year; and 1 in 2 people who smoke cigarettes regularly will eventually die as a result of their addiction.

The most common causes of death are cancer, particularly of the lung and mouth; Chronic Obstructive Pulmonary Disease (COPD) and other lung disease; heart disease; stroke; and other circulatory disease. It is estimated that on average cigarette smokers die around 10 years younger than non-smokers.

What does tobacco contain and what does smoking do to my body?

Tobacco contains over 4,000 chemical compounds which are present either in gas form, or as tiny particles, many of which are toxic to the body. Around 50 of these compounds can cause cancer including:

▶ carbon monoxide (also found in car exhaust fumes & faulty gas appliances) which reduces the amount of oxygen in the blood by taking its place. This means your lungs won't work as efficiently as those of non-smokers

▶ tar which stays inside your lungs, making your breathing tubes narrower and reducing your protection against infection. It is a sticky brown substance which also stains your fingers, teeth and hair.

▶ Cyanide (a poison used in the gas chambers), arsenic (which is rat poison), DDT and dieldrin (insecticides), methanol (rocket fuel), acetone (nail varnish remover) and formaldehyde (used for preserving dead bodies) are amongst some of the others.

So what are the health costs?

The NHS spends roughly £2.7 billion each year on treating smoking related disease of one sort or another, which is a hefty amount of money. Within this envelope of money costs for consultations with your GP, hospital admissions and prescriptions are included. However if the government achieved its target for reducing smoking a cost saving analysis has shown that a saving of up to £524 million could be made because of a reduction in the number of people having a heart attack or stroke. This would be a significant saving of public money.

In terms of lost productivity there is a significant benefit to be made which could realise a net benefit of up to £2.3 - £2.7 billion if all workplaces in England were made completely smoke free. About 34 million days are lost each year in England and Wales from sickness and ill health caused by smoking, which is a colossal amount.

In the face of all these facts and figures it is hard to justify continuing to smoke on both a health and an economic basis. So, if you are a smoker, are you ready to give up yet? Surely it is the only sensible thing to do! It's your life so why not take a massive positive step to reducing your risk of further problems now, and decide to quit?

If not, what else needs to happen in order for you to make that decision to quit??

A great way of reinforcing what a fantastic decision it was to quit smoking is to put the money for each packet of cigarettes into a piggy bank and save all the money up. At the end of a year when you come to empty it you could have saved enough money to go on the holiday of a lifetime, buy an engagement ring, buy a new sofa or anything else you have set your mind on.

OK, so let's look at how both your health and your lifestyle could improve if you gave up smoking. You will:

► Reduce your risk of developing smoking related illnesses, disability or death

► Reduce your risk of getting gangrene or needing amputation of a limb caused by problems with your circulation, especially if you are diabetic

► Improve your chances of getting pregnant and also of having a healthy baby if you do become pregnant

► Improve your breathing and general level of fitness

► Enjoy your food much more as your taste buds recover

► Protect the health of those around you, as well as improve your health, by not exposing them to second-hand smoke

► Reduce your children's chances of suffering from glue ear or asthma as they will not be passive smokers

Apart from those considerations your lifestyle will also change:

▶ You will have more money – you could save as much as several hundred pounds each month, depending on how heavily you smoke

▶ You won't smell of stale cigarette smoke

▶ The condition of your teeth and skin will improve which may also

▶ Help you feel more confident in social situations

▶ Your home won't smell of stale smoke, especially if you redecorate, as your walls won't get stained by nicotine

▶ You are less likely to have a fire at home so you will be living in a safer environment

▶ Within 1 year of quitting smoking, your risk of heart attack/stroke will be the same as that of a non-smoker

Looking at the dramatic improvements that you could make to your life can be really motivating as it isn't easy, for many people, to give up smoking. However reminding yourself that the effects of smoking on your body are pretty horrible, and that you can also cause this effect on people you live with from passive smoking, can help you stay motivated to stay off the cigarettes. It is not an attractive habit – your fingers, teeth and hair can get stained yellow from the nicotine, you get more wrinkles, constantly smell of stale smoke, etc – and it also costs you quite a bit of money each year.

Just think how great life would be if you stopped smoking! You would feel great, look great, smell great, be healthier and have more money into the bargain! And you are more likely to live longer too!

How fantastic would that be?
Worth thinking about?
Worth aiming for?
So what are you waiting for then?

First steps

I would recommend working with a trained adviser or healthcare professional to support you through the process, as well as finding someone in your personal life to support you through it too. You will have quite a tough time so why make things more difficult for yourself than you have to? Research shows that you are twice as likely to be successful in quitting if you have the help of a health professional.

The NHS offers free local support and advice that really works. They can also give you patches or gum to manage your cravings and help you to overcome your cravings. Using the patches or gum will increase your likelihood of giving up successfully by up to four times.

If you want more information and help contact the NHS Smoking Helpline on 0800 022 4332 or ask your GP or Practice Nurse for more information and support.

Psychological Well-Being

What about STRESS!

Research evidence is beginning to recognise that, for some people, prolonged episodes of stress may contribute to high blood pressure. We cannot measure stress easily which makes this area quite complex to research. However, stress can affect the heart by releasing certain chemicals or hormones – cortisol and adrenaline - that increase your blood pressure and can also increase your likelihood of developing a clot in your arteries.

Stress can increase the production of these hormones which prepare the body to react to a new challenge. You may have heard reference to the 'flight or fight' response of the body, and this is in essence what your body is preparing for. Over the centuries, if you were facing a dangerous or challenging situation such as being confronted by a bear or going into battle (or a hoodie with a knife!) this was a very useful response as it diverted blood to the areas of the body that you would need to 'fight or run for it (flight)' but in our modern westernised society you have different challenges to face, which are not necessarily immediate or obviously 'dangerous'. So if you are under pressure at work this may be for a prolonged period of time. This is when it can affect your blood pressure adversely.

Stress can also affect your state of mind and make you rely on quick fixes, rather than taking long term action to deal with the stress and prevent it building up. This can take the form of encouraging less healthy behaviours such as:

- over-eating
- smoking
- drinking too much alcohol
- taking recreational drugs.

You may also not sleep well at night which will also affect your state of mind too, and you may start to wake up early in an anxious state and not be able to get back to sleep. This also means that it discourages you from spending time on healthy behaviours such as physical activity or relaxation time.

It is important to identify the things that cause you stress, recognise when they might be affecting your health, and take action to reduce or avoid the stress so it does not affect your health.

One of the key factors that research has shown is that people are more likely to feel stressed if they feel that they have little or no control over their work, but have a lot of demands and targets placed on them to achieve. Research has also shown that people in manual jobs are more likely to be in stressful situations at work. Therefore the more you can do to control your work environment and objectives the more likely you are to have less stress. If you are able to take more control over this and influence your work targets and objectives the less likely you are to work in a stressed state of mind.

Relaxation

Relaxation is possibly one of the most important keys to health and well-being. It is an antidote to stress (which is known to contribute to disease, as has been discussed in the previous section). When we relax we give our bodies an opportunity to unwind which helps us 'recharge our batteries'. Using a car analogy, if you rev the engine a lot it will heat up and make a loud noise but if you take your foot off the accelerator pedal and let it idle it will take a while to drop down to the idling speed and a much quieter noise. Our bodies are not dissimilar and we need to allow that time to get back to our resting state.

As we already know relaxing gives our hearts a rest by slowing our heart rates. It reduces our blood pressure, decreases muscle tension and increases blood flow to the muscles. It also slows our breathing rate, which reduces our need for oxygen.

As a result of relaxing many people feel that they have:

⇨ more energy
⇨ better quality sleep
⇨ better problem-solving abilities
⇨ greater efficiency
⇨ an enhanced immunity
⇨ more even emotion (therefore less anger, anxiety, frustration and crying)
⇨ less headaches and pain

Taking time to relax is very important and you should make it one of your priorities, if you do not do so already. One of the biggest points to take on board is that we need to make time to do it, and sometimes that means giving ourselves permission to do just that. It is very easy to let it slip down the list of our priorities and become lost in the myriad of lesser priorities that we often never get round to doing.

So, STOP, and DO NOTHING! How does that feel?

Start by taking short relaxation breaks frequently throughout the day and just do nothing from time to time. Restful pauses will help you reset and recharge your energy levels, and rest is the basis for activity. Don't feel guilty if, when you get home from work you like to just sit and listen to music or let yourself float off into a nice space for a while. There is nothing wrong with doing this but we often don't give ourselves permission to do it as we feel we should be 'getting on with something more important'.

Take some deep breaths and concentrate on your breathing and how you feel when you take slow even breaths. How does it feel when air flows into your lungs (inflate every corner of them), and then out again? Try and concentrate on keeping your breathing rhythmic and steady for a few minutes and notice that natural rhythm – much like listening and watching the waves washing up and down the beach. As you concentrate on your breathing let the minutiae of the day, and any cares you have, wash away out of your mind and stay suspended in a trance-like state for 15 minutes or so to allow your body to re-energise and invigorate itself.
Notice how this feels and how your body has changed as a result of you relaxing it.

This is just one of the techniques you can train yourself to do which will help you relax. There are a whole load of ways to relax and techniques to learn if you feel you need more structured ways of learning to unwind and developing your abilities to relax, such as learning to meditate (which is a very powerful tool), listening to relaxing music or a guided meditation CD, going for walks especially if you are able to walk in the countryside or on a beach or coastal path and many other things. Just lying down and resting for 5 minutes can be refreshing, or having a 'power nap' and stacking some zzzzzzz for 20 minutes. Many people find that taking vigorous exercise helps them to unwind and relax. It is a question of finding out for yourself what works for you, and you may need to try a variety of things until you settle on what works well for you.

I could write pages and pages about relaxation, and all that it encompasses but there is not room in this book to do that. However, there are numerous places to find out more about relaxation techniques, and the internet would be a rich source to explore. The self-help section in your local bookshop would be another place to get ideas and inspiration from.

Your fitness or leisure centre will also have information about what classes or courses are available locally for you to access, and many people go on weekend breaks or holidays completely geared to relaxing, such as yoga, and meditation holidays or retreats. Why not speak to your local travel agent and see what they have to offer, if it appeals to you?

You may also have a spiritual centre near you or other local resources which you could find out about from your local Tourist Office.

Sleep

On average we spend about 30% of our lives asleep, unless we are people like Margaret Thatcher who seemed to thrive on very little sleep. For centuries sleep has been regarded as a simple shut down of activities although we had little idea why we needed it or why we spend so much of our lives having it. More recently we have a better understanding of sleep and appreciate that it is a complex process of organised physiological and behavioural states.

It is, therefore, very important to get a good night's sleep. This means ideally getting at least seven to eight hours sleep each night, certainly at least more than five hours. We have natural rhythms in our bodies called circadian rhythms which used to be associated with the natural 24 hour cycle of light and dark and as part of the daily cycle we need to allow our bodies time to rest and relax. If we ignore that need it is not only dangerous but unsustainable because our immune system and physical and mental performance are all affected by sleep and these circadian rhythms.

Over more recent years quite a few people see sleep as a bit of a waste of time and there has been a tendency to use light to greater effect to lengthen working hours. Coupled with using caffeine and nicotine as stimulants during the day and sedatives such as hypnotics and alcohol at night people are pushing themselves more, upsetting their circadian rhythms, and then having to cope with the resulting tiredness. This should plainly be avoided wherever possible, especially if it becomes a habit. Unfortunately in the UK it has become the accepted thing to work long hours and all too frequently managers foster a working environment where employees feel there is great kudos in being first in in the morning and last out at night . Productivity often falls off if long hours become the norm, and therefore this work culture should be decried and discouraged as much as possible.

People's work/life balance are all too often dictated by this type of culture and as a health coach I frequently work with people to redress the imbalance and work with individuals to find ways of bringing work more in line so that there is time in the evening to give one's personal life plenty of time to indulge and enjoy, and enable people to completely switch off from work pressures or worries. This also helps them get a good night's sleep too, which is essential for maintaining good health.

Managers and leaders play an important role in keeping their workforce healthy but sadly, all too many of them fail to acknowledge and uphold that role in the UK.

Research indicates that deep sleep, otherwise known as REM, or rapid eye movement, sleep is the most useful sleep and that any disruption of REM sleep can affect our memory and learning abilities.

If people are sleep restricted to 3-5 hours over 7 consecutive days their vigilance and performance are affected and drop. If this continues for any length of time it seems that the brain can adapt to chronic sleep deprivation although there is a marked decline in their cognitive performance and the people themselves are not likely to be aware of this.

Deprivation of sleep can also lead to lower immune defences, thought to be as a result of a rise in the blood level of a substance called cortisol. For example people who are short of sleep often catch the common cold more frequently. Sleep deprivation and prolonged psychological stress or anxiety raise cortisol levels which dampens our immune system and puts our blood pressure up. There is a definite association between sleep deprivation and high blood pressure. Cat naps can be good for you too – does a cat look stressed?

Tips for getting a good night's sleep:

⇨ Don't eat or drink alcohol late

⇨ Have a warm drink before you go to bed

⇨ Have a routine and follow it (eg close the curtains, lock the door, turn out the lights, etc.)

⇨ Read a book, or do something else that is quiet and calming before going to bed

Maintain a balance between work, play and your health.

Remember, your personal life, relationships and career make up the whole person that is you. You are more than just someone who has high blood pressure.

The following pages on Managing your Mind and Keeping Calm have been generously contributed by Damian Edwards, Senior Cognitive Behavioural Trainer and Director of Training at HDM Medical.

Managing Your Mind

In this Section, you will already have read how the connection between stress, attitude and blood pressure is still a matter for research. Yet, from a common sense point of view as well as at a clinical level, you might understand that as stress levels rise blood pressure rises with it. This happens because stress causes the body to release a flood of hormones which temporarily push blood pressure up preparing the body for 'fight or flight'. These sudden surges of high blood pressure may or may not cause long-term high blood pressure but the damage caused by the surge can strain your blood vessels and heart in just the same way.

So what can you do to avoid these stressed up spikes in blood pressure and gain better control of your mind and mood? Given that everyday life is full of all kinds of challenges, how can you remain in charge of how you feel and avoid becoming a victim of circumstance? What attitude can you adopt that is most protective of your heart, your health and your future?

The good news is that you simply do not have to live your life as a victim of circumstance. The news or the neighbours, the weather or your workmates are not meant to dictate your levels of health and happiness. Regardless of the circumstances outside of you, the fact is that how you feel is completely under your own control.

Of course it is a common misunderstanding to imagine that outside events make you feel the way you feel inside. You may say:

'The traffic today has really wound me up!' or 'The kids are getting on my nerves!'

When you imagine that other people's behaviour and arbitrary external events dictate your mood, you are thinking like a victim. To take charge of your stress levels and manage your mind it is necessary to let go of blaming outside factors. The secret is to realise how your OPINIONS about what happens are the real culprits when it comes to causing you stress.

The idea of blaming everyone and everything else for your moods may seem appealing but it actually weakens you. Your power to be healthy and happy lies in accepting responsibility for your own thoughts and, though often it might seem like everyone and everything else is responsible for your mood, in truth you are in charge of your own thoughts.

Consider how your responses to situations vary according to whether you are tired, hungry or just plain grumpy! Imagine if someone made a critical remark aimed at you. How would you feel? Hurt? Amused? Angry? Or unconcerned? Would it depend on who said it? Would it make a difference if you were already feeling low? The fact is that the same external event can create various reactions because how you feel is not dependent on what happens but instead it is dependent YOU and on your OPINION about what happens.

For example, in reaction to a hurtful remark, you might make yourself angry with thoughts like:

'He only said that to hurt me.'

'She really hates me'.

'No-one cares how I feel'.

Alternatively, you could be less concerned if you thought:

'She only said because she's jealous'.

'She only said that because she's tired'.

'He didn't mean that nastily. He's just a bit wound up.'

If you look closely at the first set of examples – the ones that make you angry - you can see how the opinions that cause a lot of stress are sometimes over-exaggerated, mostly irrational and often untrue. These thoughts are simply bad habits learnt from negative experiences; sometimes your upset can seem to teach you horrible lessons about life and damage your self-image. As a result, you can carry negative beliefs about experiences ('you can't trust anyone' or 'If it can go wrong, it will') and negative opinions about yourself ('I'm too slow to understand', 'I'll never be any good at it').

If you are not careful, these irrational opinions can remain unexamined and unchanged, leading you down a path full of stress and high blood pressure. You can end up sounding like a grumpy old man or woman complaining about how wet the rain is! The important point this: that kind of cynicism and self-deprecation is not just harmful to your mental health, it can also contribute to higher levels of stress and elevated blood pressure.

Yet fortunately, you can change your opinions and so change the way you experience the world, reducing your stress levels and your blood pressure along with it. You can achieve this simply by taking the old habit of automatically thinking negatively and swap it with a conscious effort to adopt more positive opinions about the world and yourself. You may already do this to help your friends when they seem stressed. If someone was facing redundancy or a divorce, you might encourage them to look at the situation differently by saying:

'Try not to see it as the end of the world, look at it as a new beginning'. You might encourage a tearful mother at a wedding by saying: 'Don't think of it as losing a daughter, think of it as gaining a son'.

This 'change of opinion' technique is something you probably do automatically for others, yet you could also easily start to do it consciously for yourself. If you have ever wondered how some people seem to manage stress better than you, this is their secret! Indeed, learning to let go of old, unhelpful opinions like this is a useful form of mental 'self-defence' against the 'slings and arrows' of everyday life!
Of course you may not want to stop blaming everything and everyone else for how stressed you feel. You may not want to agree that you create your own state of mind because you do not fancy that responsibility. Yet if you suffer from high blood pressure, you could benefit massively from simply adopting this one principle of 'Opinion Exchange'. By replacing harmful opinions with more helpful beliefs you are addressing the (often irrational) ideas that decide whether life is a vicious or a virtuous circle and whether your stress levels are high or low.

With just this one simple strategy, you can take charge of your own stress levels and avoid becoming a 'helpless victim' of circumstance. As you learn to think for yourself, instead of accepting negative opinions that others may have foisted upon you, you liberate your mind with a daily good habit that can ease the strain on your mind - and your body.

Keeping Calm

Suppose that your brain is like a radio, a receiver for all kinds of transmissions. Then imagine that the people around you and the events that occur are like transmissions from different radio stations – some will be upbeat, some will be downbeat, some will lift your mood whilst others could cause you a banging headache. When you tune into a station on a normal radio at home or in the car, you would usually choose a station that plays music you enjoy, rather than the ones that give you a headache! If we accept that life transmits all kinds of channels – some good and some not so good – the trick is learning how to 'tune out' the noise and 'tune in' to the music. This kind of 'mental tuning' is fundamentally what makes the difference between negative and positive mental health.

Consider the example of a girl – call her Sue - who has been stood up for a blind date. Having heard nothing from her date since he let her down and unable to raise him on the phone, what kind of 'transmissions' is Sue likely to hear? Bitter friends might tell her that 'all men are pigs!' and Sue might feel angry if she believes them; some might point out that he could have had an accident, at which she might feel concerned. Hoping to bolster Sue's self-esteem, helpful friends might scoff: 'Well, it's his loss!' On the other hand, less tactful mates might clumsily ask: 'Do you think he did turn up for the blind date, saw you and then left?' How might Sue feel then?!

As well as these 'outside transmissions', Sue will also be subject to her own 'internal transmissions' – the thoughts that she has about what happened to her Blind Date. Ironically, many of those thoughts are transmissions that other people have previously implanted in her head, so Sue could be thinking 'He probably did see me and leave, I'm so fat!' because a critical parent or cruel boyfriend convinced her that she was unattractive. Or perhaps the constant transmissions from the media, with images of stick-thin models, have made Sue believe that she is far from perfect, so she ends up thinking: 'No-one will ever fancy me!'

What is important to notice here is how Sue ends up feeling and – most importantly - how directly Sue's feelings are affected by which 'transmission' she tunes in to. Feeling concerned that he might have had an accident, feeling humiliated by apparent rejection or even being relieved by a 'lucky escape' – all of these reactions are totally dependent on the thoughts in Sue's head, not what happened on the date itself.

When 'stressful' things occur – such as losing a wallet, getting stuck in traffic, breaking something precious or being abused by another driver – how you feel is up to you. You choose which 'station' your brain tunes in to. With the example of cheeky or abusive drivers, it is common to feel 'justifiably annoyed' but is that annoyance doing you any good? In terms of your blood pressure, definitely not! When adrenalin pumps into your blood because you are angry, it is a fuel that needs burning up. If you run away from danger or fight off an assailant, then the fuel is burnt. If, however, you are just sitting in the car fuming, then the adrenalin turns into sticky fatty globules that can contribute to the narrowing of your arteries and directly affect your heart and blood pressure. Is that what you want? It is enough that some cheeky driver cuts in front of you but now you are letting that driver make you ill!

The solution is not to get out of the car and burn up the adrenaline by beating the other driver up! Not only is that illegal and dangerous but the ensuing stress will just raise your blood pressure even more! Besides, there are far too many bad drivers on the road and you do not have the time or energy to fight them all! The best way to burn up your adrenaline is healthy exercise of a type that is suited to your current medical condition and something that you enjoy. Yet the real solution here is not to get adrenalised in the first place – so how do you do that?

Again, the key here is which thoughts you choose to tune in to. If you choose indignant thoughts like 'He had no right to do that. He could have killed me!', then unsurprisingly you will feel indignant. If you choose thoughts that pressurise you into doing something such as 'I can't let him get away with that – I'll show him!' then (you guessed it!) you will feel pressurised into doing something. So what 'internal tune' can you choose to listen to that would help you keep calm?

As it happens, there are dozens of ways to view other people's behaviour that would allow you to avoid stress. You could imagine that the driver is rushing to the hospital or that they are late for a crucial job interview. You could suppose that the driver has just picked up a hire car and is used to driving in another country (this is especially true near airports). Or you could just look at the driver's manoeuvre and simply ask yourself one question: 'Have I ever done that?' – chances are that the answer is a resounding YES!

Of course these thoughts are not necessarily accurate – it is actually less likely that the driver is rushing to the hospital and more likely that he is just being pushy. But does it matter if you are right or wrong? Would you rather think that you are right (but possibly be wrong) and make yourself ill, or can you face the idea that you might be wrong but at least you are well? There is in fact an old rhyme that sums up this choice for you. It is about a driver who pushed his way out at a junction and the verse was a jokey epitaph for his driving mistake chiselled onto a cartoon headstone: His way was right and his will was strong but he's just as dead as if he was wrong!

Making the choice of which station you listen to in your head can mean the difference between sadness and sickness or happiness and health. Tuning into more positive thoughts will not miraculously cure your heart or high blood pressure problems but it will make a difference to the amount of stress you suffer, your heart rate, your blood pressure and your overall health. The immediate difference could be just that you learn to handle 'stressful' situations more calmly and laugh more at the challenges that life throws your way. In the long-term, your blood pressure, your mental health and the quality of your life could all improve.

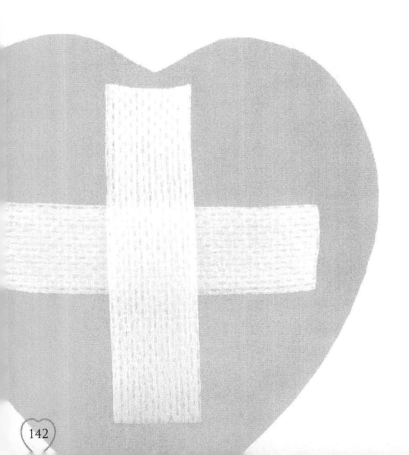

Part 3

My Blood Pressure Action Plan

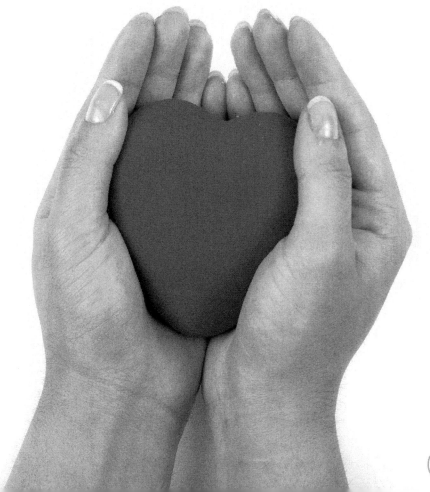

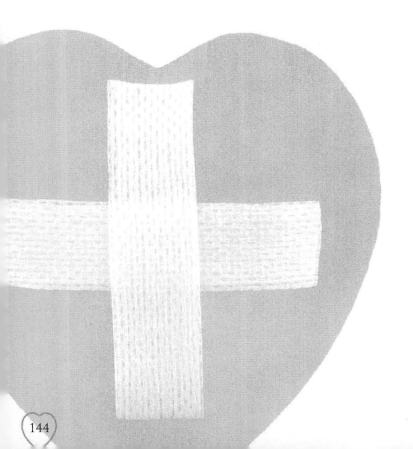

Healthy Life style Goals

Think of three things you want to achieve in the next three months. Write these down in sentences starting "I will have started exercising, or I will be taking my medication as I should!" Taking better control of your health starts here.

1. *I will* ....

....

....

....

....

....

2. *I will* ....

....

....

....

....

....

3. *I will* ....

....

....

....

....

....

Once you decide what to do, think about how to make things happen. Your personal action plan will outline the smaller steps taken to achieve your goals, and how to monitor your progress.

In a week it is realistic to complete twelve tasks that lead to what you ultimately want to do. Four tasks will relate to each goal, and as you tick them off your list, through the next week, the list for next week will begin to develop. Each week your goal becomes a reality and you are doing what you want to do.

Statement of intent

I have designed this plan to help me take control of my health. Without a plan my health condition could get worse over time and possibly affect my enjoyment of life. **Lifestyle changes and taking medication regularly may help to prevent this from happening.** *With the support of my family, friends, doctors, and health care team,* **I can** *take control of my health by setting some simple goals that* **I decide on,** *and work out how* **I can** *stick to them.*

Name...

Signed...

Date..

If it helps you to stick to your plan – ask a family member, friend or even your GP or Practice Nurse to review your plan and give you support and encouragement.

Key names and phone numbers

Doctor ....

Practice nurse ....

Practice address ....

Phone number/ after hours number ....

Self Management Coach ....

List of my health problems and medical conditions

....

....

....

....

....

....

....

....

....

....

....

My allergies or medical alerts:

....

....

....

....

....

....

....

The biggest challenge for me is:

....

....

....

....

....

....

One thing I would love to change is:

....

....

....

....

....

Any Questions I want answered:

....

....

....

....

....

....

....

....

....

....

....

....

....

....

....

....

....

....

....

....

Medicines, herbs and other remedies.

I will discuss with my pharmacist or practice team before I stop taking any of these medicines. Stopping some medicines suddenly may worsen how I feel in the long run.

Medicine 1	Date	What's it for	
How much to take and when			
Breakfast	Lunch	Dinner	Bedtime

Medicine 2	Date	What's it for	
How much to take and when			
Breakfast	Lunch	Dinner	Bedtime

Medicine 3	Date	What's it for	
How much to take and when			
Breakfast	Lunch	Dinner	Bedtime

Medicine 4	Date	What's it for

How much to take and when			
Breakfast	Lunch	Dinner	Bedtime

Medicine 5	Date	What's it for

How much to take and when			
Breakfast	Lunch	Dinner	Bedtime

Medicine 6	Date	What's it for

How much to take and when			
Breakfast	Lunch	Dinner	Bedtime

My Personal Health Goals

(Choose from the list below or add some of your own)

☐ Be more physically active

☐ Be smoke free

☐ Follow a healthy eating plan

☐ Learn about my medicines

☐ Cut down the amount of salt in my diet

☐ Learn to deal with the stress in my life

☐ Drink less alcohol

☐ Feel happier

☐ Do more things that I enjoy

☐ Lose some weight

☐ ....

☐ ....

☐ ....

☐ ....

☐ ....

☐ ....

☐ ....

☐ ....

My Major Goals

My Major Goals	How I'm going to do it	When I will achieve it

My Major Goals

My Major Goals	How I'm going to do it	When I will achieve it

Short term goals to help me achieve my major goals

My Goals	How I'm going to do it	When I will achieve it

Short term goals to help me achieve my major goals

My Goals	How I'm going to do it	When I will achieve it

Confidence Scale

Use this scale to work out how confident you are to achieve each of your goals. If you don't feel very confident, think about making your goal easier to achieve

1	2	3	4	5	6	7	8	9	10

Not at all confident   A little bit confident   Very confident

I will celebrate achieving my goals by

....

....

....

....

....

....

My Blood Pressure recordings

Date	Blood Pressure	Comments
....	....	....
....	....	....
....	....	....
....	....	....
....	....	....
....	....	....
....	....	....
....	....	....
....	....	....
....	....	....
....	....	....
....	....	....
....	....	....
....	....	....
....	....	....
....	....	....
....	....	....
....	....	....

My Blood Pressure recordings

Date	Blood Pressure	Comments

My Blood Pressure recordings

Date   Blood Pressure   Comments

....

....

....

....

....

....

....

....

....

....

....

....

....

....

....

....

....

....

....

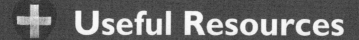

Useful Resources

Websites

Blood Pressure Association

www.bpassoc.org.uk

This association was set up for people with high blood pressure, and is a useful resource. They can give you details of your local support group and provide a lot of useful information about high blood pressure.

The British Hypertension Society

www.bhsoc.org

The British Hypertension Society provides a medical and scientific research forum to enable sharing of cutting edge research in order to understand the origin of high blood pressure and improve its treatment. An annual scientific meeting is held every September at a University Campus in the UK and Ireland.

National Institute for Health and Clinical Excellence (NICE)

www.nice.org.uk

NICE is an independent organisation responsible for providing national guidance on promoting good health and preventing and treating ill health. The hypertension guidelines can be found at: **www.nice.org.uk/CG034**

The DASH Diet
www.dashdiet.org

The DASH (Dietary Approaches to Stop Hypertension) website is very useful for giving more detailed information. The DASH diet helps to lower blood pressure by providing more key nutrients, such as potassium, calcium, and magnesium, all of which are associated with lower blood pressure. These key nutrients are boosted by including more fruits, vegetables, and low-fat or non-fat dairy in your daily diet.

The Food Standards Agency (FSA)
www.foodstandards.gov.uk

The Food Standards Agency is charged with protecting consumer interests in relation to food safety and standards. Most importantly, the Agency is entitled to make public the advice that it gives to Government ministers. This means that the Agency can be seen to act openly and independently in looking after the interests of consumers. This website provides very useful information regarding food labelling etc.

NHS Direct
www.nhsdirect.nhs.uk

NHS Direct is here for you whenever you have health worries and they have the knowledge and experience to give you real help and reassurance. Their vision is to be the national healthline, providing expert health advice, information and reassurance, using their world class telephone service and website, and to be the NHS' provider of choice for telephone and digitally delivered health services. This is always a good place to start if you need some information or advice.

Diet Chef
www.dietchef.co.uk

This diet is for anyone who says they are too busy to cook healthy food to help them lose weight. They will prepare 3 calorie controlled meals a day for you helping you to lose weight and lower your blood pressure.

Action on Smoking and Health
www.ash.org.uk

This website provides up to the minute information on key tobacco issues.

The Ramblers
www.ramblers.org.uk

The Ramblers is Britain's walking charity, working to safeguard the footpaths, the countryside and other places we go walking, and to encourage more people to take up walking. With 119,000 members in England, Scotland and Wales, we've been working for walkers for 76 years.

Walking for Health
www.whi.org.uk

Walking for Health (WfH) encourages more people to become physically active in their local communities. WfH supports the largest network of health walk schemes across England, offering regular short walks over easy terrain with trained walk leaders. WfH was established in 2000 and has stood the test of time. With over 600 local schemes, WfH contributes to improving the health of 66,000 regular walkers nationwide.

British Military Fitness

www.britmilfit.com

British Military Fitness (BMF) is the largest and longest running provider of outdoor fitness classes in the UK.

All year round, BMF runs over 400 classes a week in 105 parks across the UK. All the 500 plus instructors are serving or former members of the armed forces. Highly trained, experienced, and responsible in their approach to training. Graded by ability - beginner, intermediate or advanced – BMF delivers an invigorating outdoor workout that's right for your fitness level. BMF have over 20,000 members of all shapes and sizes, ages and backgrounds. Why not come along and experience it for yourself?

The National Trust

www.nationaltrust.org.uk

The National Trust (NT) has over 3.6 million members and 55,000 volunteers. More than 14 million people visit our pay for entry properties, while an estimated 50 million visit our open air properties. NT protects and opens to the public over 350 historic houses, gardens and ancient monuments. But it doesn't stop there. NT also look after forests, woods, fens, beaches, farmland, downs, moorland, islands, archaeological remains, castles, nature reserves, villages - for ever, for everyone. Learn new skills, meet new people, work right at the heart of amazing buildings, gardens and landscapes. Just imagine what you could do...

Crystal Waters

www.onlinefish.co.uk

Currently the demand for healthy eating is a matter for all to stop and consider as our life styles get busier and busier. The trap which we have all fallen into with the need for 'fast' ' 'junk food' ' convenience food' increases the need for the 'retailer' to provide a quick & nutritional alternative, is crucial and this is exactly what we are trying to do. This is a family run business of 10 years, which produces ALL their own smoked fish with enthusiasm and love. They use traditional methods for 90% of their products & do not use any additives or preservatives. More recently they are perfecting new and exciting methods for producing smoked fish, produced from more sustainable sources... They can send nearly all the smoked ranges through the post. The website gives a list of 'when & where to find us' if you live in East Anglia and can access one of their fresh fish stalls in a variety of markets. List of some smoked products they produce include:

Traditional Oak Smoked Undyed Kippers, Kiln Roasted Oak Smoked Whole Mackerel, Traditional Oak Smoked Kiln Roasted Mackerel Fillets, Traditional Oak Smoked Kiln Roasted Salmon, Traditional Cold Smoked Salmon to name but a few...

hdm-medical
www.hdm-medical.com
hdm-medical provides professional training for Healthcare Professionals, specialising in Cognitive Behaviour Therapy, Addictive Behaviour, Motivational Interviewing, Stress Management, Patient Self-Management and Obesity.

Sports clubs and associations

www.sports-clubs.net
This website lists many different sports and activities and gives details of how to find out more information or how/where they are in your local area. This is a very useful resource.

Books

There are a great number of books available, and different authors with different approaches suit different people. One I know that many have found helpful and have recommended is:

I Can Make You Thin, by Paul McKenna
(Bantam Press 2005; ISBN 0593050541)

Helplines

NHS Smoking Helpline: 0800 022 4332

Weight Loss Helpline: 0151 222 4737

➕ Index

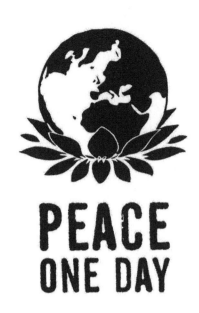

PEACE ONE DAY

Jeremy Gilley is an actor turned filmmaker, who in the late 1990s became preoccupied with questions about the fundamental nature of humanity and the issue of peace. He decided to explore these through the medium of film, and specifically, to create a documentary following his campaign to establish an annual day of ceasefire and non-violence. In 1999, Jeremy founded Peace One Day, a non-profit organisation, and in 2001 Peace One Day's efforts were rewarded when the member states of the United Nations unanimously adopted the first ever day of global ceasefire and non-violence on 21 September annually – Peace Day.

In 2007 Jeremy and Peace One Day ambassador Jude Law travelled to Afghanistan to spearhead a campaign that has resulted in 4.5 million children being vaccinated against polio in hitherto unreachable areas as a result of Peace Day agreements by all parties to conflict in the region in 2007/8/9.

In 2010, millions of people were active on Peace Day, in all 192 UN member states, and 28 organisations carried out 88 humanitarian activities across 31 countries. For Peace Day 2010, in Afghanistan WHO/UNICEF/Afghan Ministry of Public Health vaccinated over 50,000 children and women in 23 locations against all vaccine-preventable diseases. They also launched a nationwide polio campaign targeting 8 million children across the country.

With the day in place Peace One Day is working to institutionalise Peace Day, making it a day that is self-sustaining. The next stepping-stone on this journey is to reach 3 billion people with the message of Peace Day by September 2012. For Peace Day 2012, Peace One Day is calling for and working towards a day of ceasefire and non-violence – a Global Truce. POD hopes that this will be the largest reduction in global violence in recorded history.

To get involved go to www.peaceoneday.org

What will you do to make peace on 21 September?

Notes

Notes

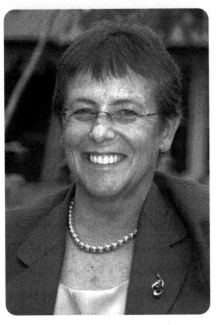

About the Author

Katy Gordon is an outstanding health care specialist, having worked as a nurse, senior manager and healthcare consultant in the NHS for over 30 years. Katy has had experience as a cardiac nurse and as a Sister on Westminster Hospital's Intensive Care Unit, in the front line for all bomb-blast injuries in London. She was also one of the key co-organisers for the medical team on the mercy flight to retrieve British hostages from Baghdad during the first Iraq War, along with Richard Branson and former UK premier Ted Heath. She is also a health coach.

Katy understands every aspect of the patient experience, from the most extreme to the most mundane, and explains complex medical questions clearly, straightforwardly and with gentle humour.

Katy herself has been diagnosed with high blood pressure, and speaks from first-hand experience as well as up-to-the-minute medical understanding.

Her advice is well worth taking.

www.katygordon.com